Keto Cha

Quick, Easy, And Mouthwatering
Chaffle Recipes
To Support Your Weight Loss And
Healthy Life.

Emily Todd

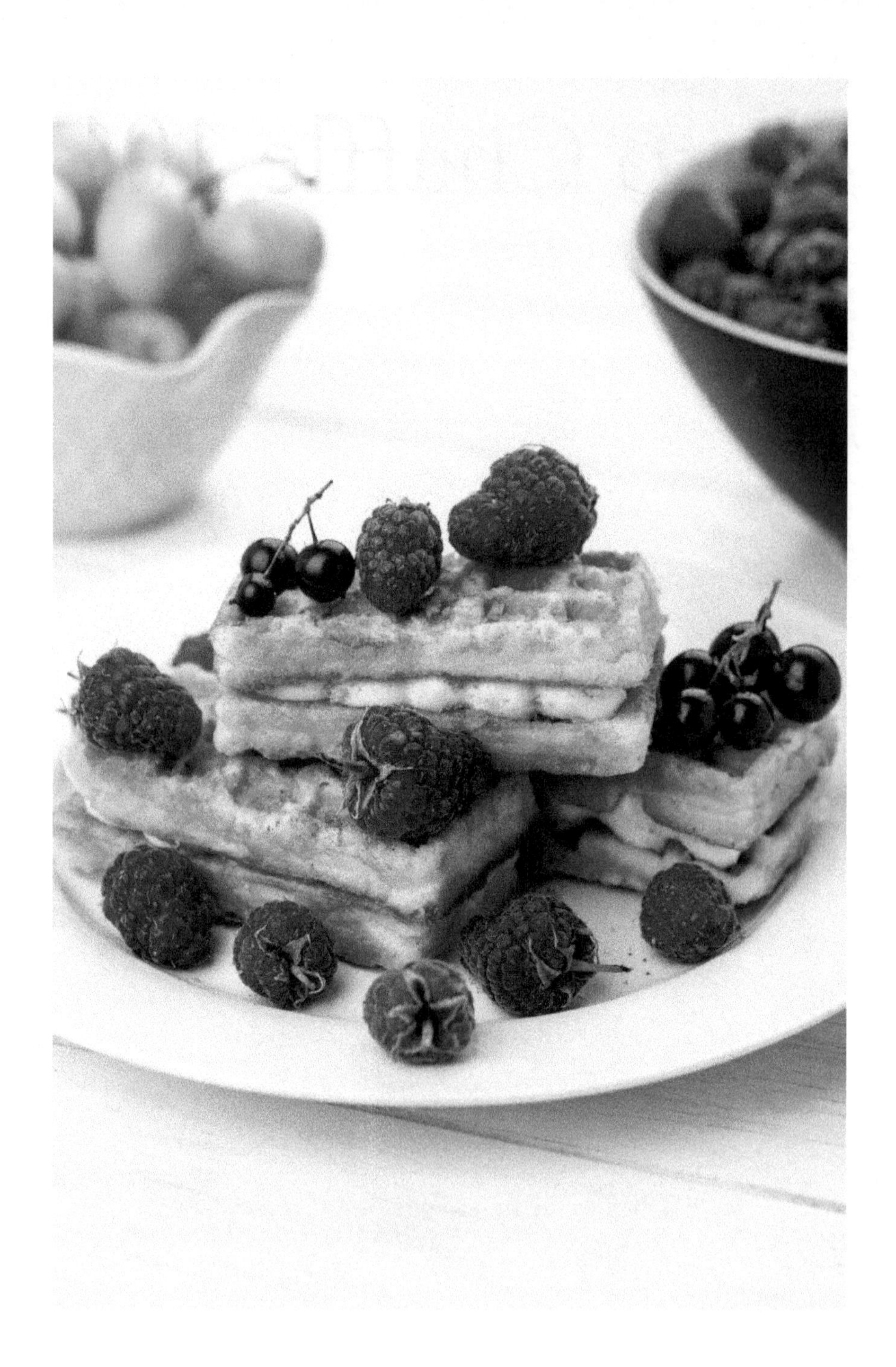

Chapter 1. Table of Contents

Introduction

Keto is the new word in weight loss. It's a very healthy eating routine that stimulates your body to burn fat instead of carbohydrates for energy.

The ketogenic diet has become popular over the past few years. This regimen is based around a metabolic state called ketosis and involves drastically reducing carbohydrate intake. During the Ketogenic diet, you will eat high amounts of fat, few carbs, and moderate amounts of protein. This causes your body to use stored fat instead of glucose to produce energy, resulting in weight loss and reduced blood sugar levels.

. It usually is used to treat various diseases or conditions such as epilepsy, diabetes, and even obesity. Once you are on this diet, you will be able to see its advantages in action and reap all the benefits it has to offer!

Eating keto chaffle can help you transition into this diet more accessible. Keto chaffles are essentially a form of a keto-friendly muffin made with high amounts of fat and low amounts of carbohydrates. They have a great taste and make a great snack or addition to any meal. Chaffles tend to be versatile and can be prepared for breakfast, lunch, or dinner.

They also make great additions to your meal plans because they are a healthy way to get in your fiber, vitamins, and minerals. Many people find it helpful to curb their appetite, so you won't feel hungry throughout the day as you typically would without them being in your diet.

When using this cookbook, you can not only enjoy these chaffles but also record all your other meals with them as well! This will support you track your progress and motivate you to make the changes that will allow you to reach your goals. You can buy this book even if you don't follow the diet by itself but still want this manual for another purpose.

Understanding the benefits of keto chaffles is one thing; having them in your own home is another! So don't hesitate; jump on board and start enjoying this fantastic way of eating today!

Besides having chaffles as your main dish, you can also add chilies, cheese, and other vegetables to make it flavorful.

Chapter 2. What Is A Chaffle, Why Chaffles Well Fit With A Keto Regime?

Chaffles (short for cheddar Chaffles) is the most recent famous nourishment in the keto world. It's nothing unexpected; the chaffle has a great deal putting it all on the line. This straightforward keto formula is fresh, brilliant dark-colored, sans sugar, low-carb, and exceptionally simple to make.

A chaffle, or cheddar Chaffle, is a keto Chaffle made with eggs and cheddar. Chaffles is turning into an exceptionally well-known keto/low-carb nibble.

A chaffle is a Chaffle yet made with a cheddar base. Its obliterated cheddar and an egg mix. Once in for a short time for logically fluffier recipes, it's a cream cheddar base instead of decimated cheddar. It's the a la mode new keto-pleasing bread since its low in carbs, and it won't spike your insulin levels, causing fat to accumulate.

The fundamentals are some combo of egg and cheddar; however, you can riff like wild-eyed from here. You can use an arrangement of cheeses, including cream cheddar, parmesan cheddar, etc. Some incorporate almond flour and flaxseed and getting ready powder and others don't.

The primary recipe for a chaffle contains cheddar, almond flour, and an egg. You consolidate the fixings in an astonish and pour it your Chaffle maker. Chaffle makers are no doubt on the rising right now after this chaffle recipe exploded a couple of days back earlier. I was to some degree suspicious from the beginning intuition there was no possibility this would turn out in the wake of joining everything and pouring the hitter over the Chaffle. Try to sprinkle the Chaffle maker generously. The Chaffle wound up exceptional, and it was firm apparently and fragile on the inside.

You can concoct a chaffle utilizing a Chaffle iron or smaller than usual Chaffle producer. The Cooking time is just a couple of moments, and on the off chance that you are cooking the chaffle right, you end up with a fresh, gooey, flavorful bread/Chaffle elective.

Chaffles is turning into somewhat of a furor with supporters of the keto diet. They're less fastidious about making than most keto bread recipes, and they're anything but difficult to customize. You can transform the fundamental formula for a chaffle into your creation, running from flavorful to sweet and anything in the middle. You can likewise change the sort of cheddar you use, delivering significant changes in the flavor and surface of the chaffle. Cheddar and mozzarella cheddar are the two most regular decisions, yet you can likewise include parmesan, cream cheddar, or whatever other cheddar that melts well.

The most fundamental clarification of a Chaffee is that it's extraordinary bread elective on the keto diet. It copies the vibe of a Chaffle. However, Keto clients have been utilizing Chaffles in a wide range of recipes, from sandwiches to sweets. There are a considerable amount of Keto Chaffle Recipes out there.

It's made with cheddar, so get it? At the point when you work cheddar and Chaffle – you get chaffle (and you additionally get enchantment.) Well enough with the back story. Since you realize what this keto nourishment is, how about we make one and let you see with your own eyes how amazing this keto Chaffle is.

Chapter 3. The Ketogenic Diet and Its Benefits

A diet that results in the production of ketone bodies by the liver is called a Ketogenic diet; it causes your system to use fat instead of carbohydrates for energy. However, it is not a high protein diet. It involves moderate protein, low carbohydrate intake, and high fat intake. The exact percentage of macronutrients varies according to your needs. Fats make up 75% of the calories you eat, making them a key component of your diet; protein makes up 30% of the calories you eat, and carbohydrates 10%.

Your system generally works with a mixture of proteins, carbohydrates, and fats. This diet eliminates carbohydrates, which causes the system's reserves to be depleted and the body to find an alternative source of energy.

Insufficient free fatty acid disintegration releases as a by-product of ketone bodies. The power supplied is fat obtained non-carbohydrate which is used by organs like the brain. As a consequence of the rapid manufacturing of ketone bodies, which makes them accumulate in the blood, ketosis develops. The manufacture and use of glucose in your system are also reduced; the protein used for power is also reduced.

The levels of glucagon and glucose are affected by Ketogenic diets. Insulin transforms glucose into glycogen that is recycled as fat, while glucagon transforms glycogen into glucose to provide your system with power. Carbs removal from the diet improves the levels of glucagon and decreases levels of insulin. This, in the end, causes liberation of an increased number of FFA and their decomposition in the liver that results in the manufacturing of ketone bodies and induces the ketosis state.

The diet is, in a way, identical to starvation, with the distinction being that food is eaten in one. The metabolic impacts that come about and the adjustments experienced in famine are approximately the same as those experienced during the diet. There has been an extensive study of the reaction to complete hunger, probably more so than the diet on its own. That's why the vast bulk of the information described is derived from the analyses of fasting individuals. There are few exceptions, but the diet's metabolic impacts are similar to those that occur during starvation. The reactions in ketosis as a result of carb restriction are the same as the reactions seen with hunger. In this regard, protein and fat amounts are not that important.

Considering how carbs are not wanted in this diet, it may leave you wondering how much is needed for daily sustenance by your system. The body undergoes at least three significant adjustments when carbs are taken away from the diet to preserve the little glucose and protein it has. The principal adjustment is a general change in power source to FFA from glucose in most of your organs. This change spares the small quantity of glucose accessible to power the brain. In the leukocytes, erythrocytes, and bone marrow that continue to use glucose, the second adaptation happens. These tissues break down glucose partly to lactate and pyruvate that go to the liver and are transferred back to glucose to avoid the depletion of accessible glucose reserve. Therefore, this issue doesn't end in a significant decrease of glucose in your system and can be ignored in terms of the carbs need of the body. The third, and likely the most important, adjustment happens in your body, which, by the third week of continuous ketosis, transforms to the use of ketones for 75% of the power demands instead of getting from carbs. Since the brain continuously depletes glucose in the body, the regular carbohydrate demands are all that we need to bother ourselves with.

Your brain uses about 100 g of glucose daily in normal conditions. This implies that any diet that is based on fewer than 100 g of carbs daily will cause ketosis, the level of which depends on how many carbs are consumed. That is, the fewer carbs eaten, the greater the ketosis. Eating carbs below 100 grams will result in ketosis. With the continued adaptation of the brain to the use of ketones for power and the glucose demands of your system decline, fewer carbs should be absorbed so as to sustain the ketosis state.

There is no one-size-fits-all when it comes to how much of your total calorie requirement you should derive from carbs. Some nutritionists advise that people keep it in the low end, which is five percent, but it is not necessarily good advice as the exact amount depends on your system. To get the right amount for you will have to rely on the trial-and-error method. Select a percentage and see how it feels for you. With fats and protein, just like in carbs, there is no exact amount for everyone. It all depends on you, but seventy-five percent is an excellent addition to start off.

There is no space to' cheat' your diet here. You should follow it completely, as even one meal that does not follow its rules can slow down your advancement for about a week as your body is withdrawn from ketosis. Always make sure you've eaten enough so that you will not be tempted to have a snack that could ruin all you've been working for.

Keto Diet Benefits

We have a lot of benefits to starting a Ketogenic diet, be it in terms of weight, experience, or to improve your health!

Effective in Fighting Epilepsy

The primary goal of this diet, introduced in Antiquity, was to fight against epilepsy. The ketones may affect anti-convulsion, but to date, it is not possible to say why they have this effect on the body.

Without going too far into the scientific part, ketone bodies would have an impact on the concentrations of glutamate and GABA (Gamma-Amino Butyric Acid). Glutamate is the primary excitatory neuro mediator of the central nervous system, and GABA the primary inhibitory neuro mediator. This would explain why the Ketogenic diet has such essential effects on people with epilepsy. But I don't want to lose you with my scientific explanations; you can do your own research if the subject interests you.

Effective in Weight Loss

Your body's source of energy in the Ketogenic diet is fat, either from food or stored by your body. This, therefore, has advantages: the level of insulin, a hormone that stores fat, drops very significantly. This means that your body will become more efficient at burning fat.

Effective in Type I or Type II Diabetes

Diabetes results in a problem in the metabolism of carbohydrates. The diet is, therefore, naturally add to relieve the signs and symptoms in a person with diabetes, whether for type I or type II diabetes. In fact, whether the problem is a defect in insulin production or insulin resistance, the Ketogenic diet will make it possible to get around the problem.

When you are Keto-adapted, your blood sugar drops sharply because you only eat foods low in carbohydrates. The Ketogenic diet can therefore allow you to control your blood sugar, which can be very effective in managing your diabetes. The Ketogenic diet will allow you to reduce your insulin levels to healthy and stable values.

Effective in People with Alzheimer's

Excuse me in advance, but in this part, we will tackle a scientific "hair" side to explain the benefits of the Ketogenic diet in the treatment of Alzheimer's disease.

The Ketogenic diet is successful in the treatment of neurodegenerative diseases like Alzheimer's because it aims to increase the enzymes of mitochondrial metabolism. Clearly, this would develop more energy in the brain and therefore improve cognitive efficiency.

In addition to all this, the Ketogenic diet would have a role in protecting against oxidative stress, and therefore would be preventive and effective against cell death. This would consequently limit brain degeneration.

Improves Concentration

Ketones are an excellent source of fuel for the brain. As you decrease your carbohydrate intake, you avoid blood sugar spikes, which often appear after meals. This allows your body to prevent focusing on eliminating carbohydrates and on concentrate on the activity you are doing.

Good for Cholesterol

As said above, if you pay attention to the quality of the fats you consume, you will see an improvement in cholesterol: you will see your good cholesterol (HDL: High-Density Lipoprotein) increase, while your bad cholesterol (LDL: Low-Density Lipoprotein) will decrease.

You will also notice an improvement in triglyceride levels, as well as an improvement in blood pressure. Blood pressure problems are usually caused by being overweight, and the Ketogenic diet is intended to cause weight loss and therefore reduce blood pressure problems.

Chapter 4. Tips for Making the Perfect Chaffles/ How to Make Chaffles

A chaffle is a keto Chaffle. It's called a chaffle because one of the main ingredients is shredded cheese, hence the chaffle instead of Chaffle because chaffles are cheese Chaffles. Pretty cool, right?

Chaffles are typically made of a flour-based batter, but a chaffle is made of eggs and cheese. It sounds odd, but it works!

Chaffles are a perfect way for those on the keto diet to get their Chaffle fix. They're also a perfect way to eat less carbs while still eating what you want! Even though it is a modified version. There are also countless chaffle ingredient variations.

How to Make Chaffles?

Equipment and Ingredients

Making chaffles requires five basic steps and nothing more than a Chaffle maker for flat chaffles and a Chaffle bowl maker for chaffle bowls.

To make chaffles, you will need two required ingredients –eggs and cheese. My favorite cheeses are cheddar cheese or mozzarella cheese. These melt easily, making them the go-to for most recipes. Meanwhile, always ensure that your cheeses are finely grated or thinly sliced for use.

Now, to make a normal chaffle:

- First, preheat your Chaffle maker until sufficiently hot.
- Meanwhile, in a cup, mix the egg with cheese on hand until well mixed.
- Open the iron, pour in a quarter or half of the mixture, and close.
- Cooking the chaffle for 5 to 7 minutes or until it is crispy.
- Transfer the chaffle to a plate and allow cooling before serving.

11 Tips to Make Chaffles

1. Preheat Well: Yes! It sounds obvious to preheat the Chaffle iron before use. However, preheating the iron moderately will not make your chaffles as crispy as you will like. The easiest way to preheat before Cooking is to ensure that the iron is very hot.
2. Not-So-Cheesy: Would you choose to make your chaffles less cheesy? Then, use mozzarella cheese.

3. Not-So Eggy: If you aren't comfortable with the smell of eggs in your chaffles, try using egg whites instead of egg yolks or whole eggs.
4. To Shred or Slice: Many recipes call for shredded cheese when making chaffles, but I find sliced cheeses to offer crispier pieces. While I stick with mostly shredded cheese for convenience's sake, be at ease to use sliced cheese in the same quantity. When using sliced cheeses, arrange two to four pieces in the Chaffle iron, top with the beaten eggs, and some cheese slices. Cover and Cooking until crispy.
5. Shallower Irons: For better crisps on your chaffles, use shallower Chaffle irons as they Cooking easier and faster.
6. Layering: Don't fill up the Chaffle iron with too much batter. Work between a quarter and a half cup of total ingredients per batch for correctly done chaffles.
7. Patience: It is a virtue even when making chaffles. For the best results, allow the chaffles to sit in the iron for 5 to 7 minutes before serving.
8. No Peeking: 7 minutes isn't too much of a time to wait for the outcome of your chaffles, in my opinion. Opening the iron and checking on the chaffle before it is done stands you a worse chance of ruining it.
9. Crispy Cooling: For better crispiness, I find that allowing the chaffles to cool further after transferring to a plate aids a lot.
10. Easy Cleaning: For the best cleanup, wet a paper towel and wipe the iron's inner parts while still warm. Kindly note that the iron should be warm but not hot!
11. Brush It: Also, use a clean toothbrush to clean between the iron's teeth for a thorough cleanup. You can also use a dry, rough sponge to clean the iron while it is still warm

Chapter 5. How to Clean Your Chaffle Maker

Make sure that it is not hot before you clean the Chaffle or chaffle maker.

But clean it as soon as it is cool enough.

- Use a damp cloth or paper towel for wiping away the crumbs.
- Soak up the excess oil drips on your grid plates.
- Rub the exterior with a damp cloth or paper towel.
- Whisk a few drops of Cooking oil on the batter to remove the stubborn batter drips. Allow it to sit for a few minutes. Wipe it away after this.
- You can wash the Cooking plates in warm soapy water. Rinse them clean.
- Ensure that the Chaffle maker is completely dry before storing it.

Chaffle Maker Maintenance Tips

Remember these simple tips, and your Chaffle maker will serve you for a long time.

- Always read the instruction manual before you use it for the first time.
- Only a light Cooking oil coating is required for nonstick Chaffle makers.
- Grease the grid with only a little amount of oil if you see the Chaffles sticking.
- Never use metal or sharp tools to scrape off the batter or to remove the Cooking Chaffles. You may end up scratching the surface and damaging it.
- Do not submerge your electric Chaffle maker in water.

Tips On How To Properly Store Keto Chaffles To Keep Them Fresh.

Here are some things you can do to ensure optimal freshness for your chaffles.

Freezing your chaffles for storage

You may want to consider freezing your chaffles to preserve freshness. Freezing your keto chaffle ensures it stays fresh and makes it easier to travel with them. If you're going on a trip, simply freeze them before you go and pack them in a cooler or insulated lunch box. Once you get to your destination and open up the chaffles, they will be thawed and ready to eat.

Using a Ziploc freezer bag

A good Ziploc bag is a perfect way to store keto chaffles for later use.

A Ziploc bag is ideal because they are reusable and non-toxic. It keeps the chaffle fresh and makes it easier to travel with. If you don't mind reusing the Ziploc bags, you can just purchase a few at once and reuse them over and over again for storing your chaffles. This way, you won't have to worry about your chaffles getting stale or moldy. The reusable Ziploc bags are also perfect because they are easy to pop in the microwave. You can easily reheat chaffle in a minimal amount of time.

When it comes to storing your keto chaffle, you want to make sure you Cooking them enough for them to be warm when eating them. If you want to reheat a chaffle in the microwave, make sure you don't eat it too much, so it doesn't go soggy.

Other ways of storing your keto chaffle include using Glad Ziploc bags or Ziploc storage bags. This will keep them fresh until they are needed.

Silicone [can] containers

Another option for storing your chaffles is by using a silicone container. Silicone containers are relatively cheap, and they can be used over and over again.

In terms of storage, silicone containers are also ideal because they seal tightly, which prevents moisture from getting in. This not only preserves your chaffle, but also keeps it fresh for the long haul.

Sealed glass containers

Other sources for purchasing sealed glass containers to store keto chaffles include Amazon and the Container Store.

The containers are ideal because they seal airtight and keep moisture out, so your chaffles are always fresh. The sealed glass container also allows you to see what's in the container, which helps when it comes to knowing when the chaffle is done Cooking.

Chapter 6. Breakfast

1. Cheese Broccoli Chaffles

Preparation Time: 5 minutes

Cooking Time: 16 minutes

Servings: 4

Ingredients:

- 1/2 cup Cooked broccoli, chopped finely
- 2 organic eggs, beaten
- 1/2 cup Cheddar cheese, shredded
- 1/2 cup Mozzarella cheese, shredded
- 2 tablespoons Parmesan cheese, grated
- 1/2 teaspoon onion powder

Directions:

1. Preheat a Chaffle iron and then grease it.
2. In a bowl, place all Ingredients and mix until well merged.
3. Set half of the mixture into preheated Chaffle iron and Cooking for about 4 minutes or until golden brown.
4. Repeat with the remaining mixture.
5. Serve warm.

Nutrition:

Calories: 112

Net Carb: 1.2g

Fat: 8.1g

Saturated Fat: 4.3g

Carbohydrates: 1.59

Sugar: 0.5g

Protein: 8.

2. Bacon and Ham Chaffle

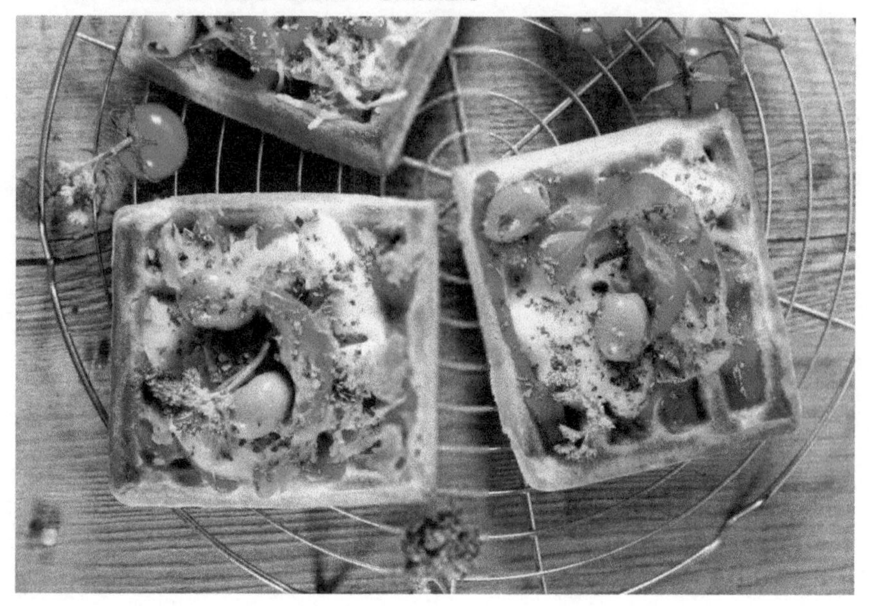

Preparation Time: 5 minutes

Cooking Time: 5 minutes

Servings: 2

Ingredients:

- 3 egg
- 1/2 cup grated Cheddar cheese
- 1 Tbsp. almond flour
- 1/2 tsp. baking powder

For the toppings:

- 4 strips Cooked bacon
- 2 pieces Bibb lettuce
- 2 slices preferable ham

- 2 slices tomato

Directions:

1. Turn on Chaffle maker to heat and oil it with Cooking spray.
2. Combine all chaffle components in a small bowl.
3. Add around 1/4 of total batter to Chaffle maker and spread to fill the edges. Close and Cooking for 4 minutes.
4. Remove and let it cool on a rack.
5. Repeat for the second chaffle.
6. Top one chaffle with a tomato slice, a piece of lettuce, and bacon strips, and then cover it with second chaffle.
7. Plate and enjoy.

Nutrition

Carbs: 5g

Fat: 60 g

Protein: 31 g

Calories: 631

3. Ham and Jalapenos Chaffle

Preparation Time: 5 minutes

Cooking Time: 9 minutes

Servings: 3

Ingredients:

- 2 Tbsp. cheddar cheese, finely grated
- 2 large eggs
- 1/2 jalapeno pepper, finely grated
- 2 ounces ham steak
- 1 medium scallion
- 2 tsp. coconut flour

Directions:

1. Set your Chaffle iron with Cooking spray and heat for 3 minutes.
2. Pour 1/4 of the batter mixture into the Chaffle iron.
3. Cooking for 3 minutes, until crispy around the edges.
4. Remove the Chaffles from the heat and repeat until all the batter is finished.
5. Once done, allow them to cool to room temperature and enjoy.
6. Shred the cheddar cheese using a fine grater.
7. Deseed the jalapeno and grate using the same grater.
8. Finely chop the scallion and ham.
9. Serve!

4. Crispy Bagel Chaffle

Preparation Time: 15 minutes

Cooking Time: 30 minutes

Servings: 1

Ingredients:

- 2 eggs
- 2 cup parmesan cheese
- 1 tsp. bagel seasoning
- 1/2 cup mozzarella cheese
- 2 teaspoons almond flour

Directions:

1. Turn on Chaffle maker to heat and oil it with Cooking spray.
2. Evenly sprinkle half of cheeses to a griddle and let them melt. Then toast for 30 seconds and leave them wait for batter.
3. Whisk eggs, other half of cheeses, almond flour, and bagel seasoning in a small bowl.
4. Pour batter into the Chaffle, Cooking for minutes.
5. Let cool for 2-3 minutes before serving.

Nutrition:

Carbs: g

Fat: 20 g

Protein: 21 g

Calories: 28 7

5. Sausage and Veggies Chaffles

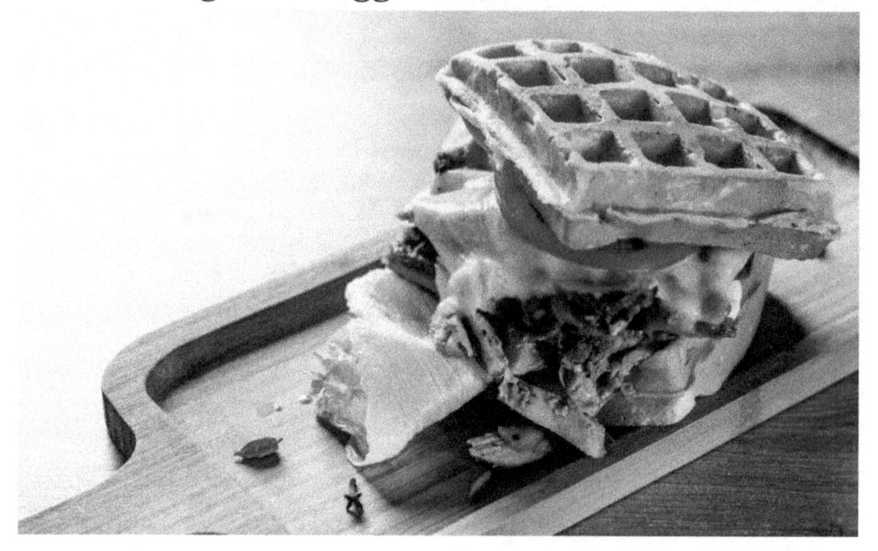

Preparation Time: 5 minutes

Cooking Time: 20 minutes

Servings: 4

Ingredients:

- 1/3 cup unsweetened almond milk
- 4 medium organic eggs
- 2 tablespoons gluten-free breakfast sausage, cut into slices
- 2 tablespoons broccoli florets, chopped
- 2 tablespoons bell peppers, seeded and chopped
- 2 tablespoons Mozzarella cheese, shredded

Directions:

1. Preheat a Chaffle iron and then grease it.
2. In a medium bowl, place the almond milk and eggs and beat well.

3. Place the remaining Ingredients: and stir to combine well.
4. Place 1/4 of the mixture into preheated Chaffle iron and Cooking for about 5 minutes or until golden brown.
5. Repeat with the remaining mixture.
6. Serve warm.

Nutrition:

Calories: 13 2

Net Carb: 1.2 g

Fat: 9.2 g

Saturated Fat: 3.5g

Carbohydrates: 1

Sugar: 0.5 g

Protein: 11.1g

Chapter 7. Brunch

6. Garlic and Thyme Lamb Chops

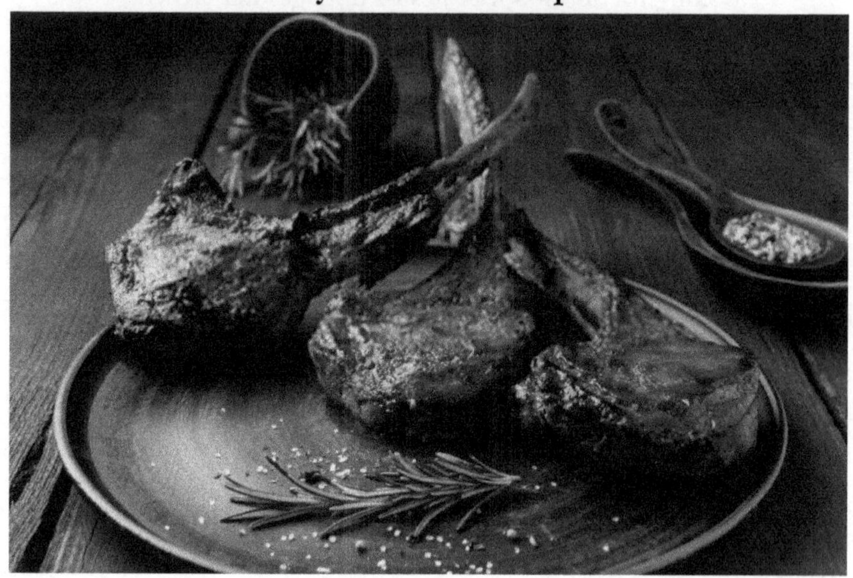

Preparation Time: 15 minutes

Cooking Time: 10 minutes

Servings: 6

Ingredients:

- 6-4 oz. Lamb chops
- 4 whole garlic cloves
- 2 thyme sprigs
- 1 tsp. Ground thyme
- 3 tbsp. Olive oil

Directions:

1. Warm-up a skillet. Put the olive oil. Rub the chops with the spices.
2. Put the chops in the skillet with the garlic and sprigs of thyme.
3. Sauté within 3 to 4 minutes and serve.

Nutrition:

Net Carbohydrates: 1 g

Protein: 14 g

Total Fats: 21 g

Calories: 252

7. Jamaican Jerk Pork

Preparation Time: 15 minutes

Cooking Time: 4 hours

Servings: 12

Ingredients:

- 1 tbsp. Olive oil
- 4 lb. Pork shoulder
- .5 cup Beef Broth
- .25 cup Jamaican Jerk spice blend

Directions:

1. Rub the roast well the oil and the jerk spice blend. Sear the roast on all sides. Put the beef broth.
2. Simmer within four hours on low. Shred and serve.

Nutrition:

Net Carbohydrates: 0 g

Protein: 23 g

Total Fats: 20 g

Calories: 282

8. Ketogenic Meatballs

Preparation Time: 15 minutes

Cooking Time: 20 minutes

Servings: 10

Ingredients:

- 1 egg
- .5 cup Grated parmesan
- .5 cup Shredded mozzarella
- 1 lb. Ground beef
- 1 tbsp. garlic

Directions:

1. Warm-up the oven to reach 400. Combine all of the fixings.
2. Shape into meatballs. Bake within 18-20 minutes. Cool and serve.

Nutrition:

Net Carbohydrates: 0.7 g

Protein: 12.2 g

Total Fats: 10.9 g

Calories: 153

Chapter 8. Lunch

9. Crab Chaffles

Preparation Time: 5 minutes

Cooking Time: 25 minutes

Servings: 6

Ingredients:

- 1 lb. crab meat
- 1/3 cup Panko breadcrumbs
- 1 egg
- 2 tbsp. fat Greek yogurt
- 1 tsp. Dijon mustard
- 2 tbsp. parsley and chives, fresh
- 1 tsp. Italian seasoning
- 1 lemon, juiced

Directions:

1. Salt, pepper to taste
2. Add the meat. Mix well.
3. Form the mixture into round patties. Cooking 1 patty for 3 minutes.
4. Remove it and repeat the process with the remaining crab chaffle mixture. Once ready, remove and enjoy warm.

10. Bacon and Egg Chaffles

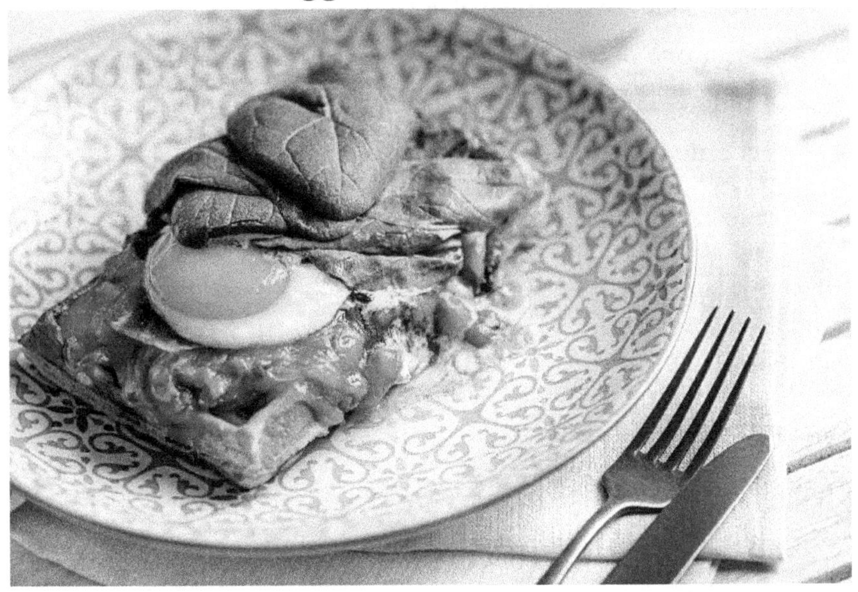

Preparation Time: 5 minutes

Cooking Time: 10 minutes

Servings: 2

Ingredients:

- 2 eggs
- 4 tsp. collagen peptides, grass-fed
- 2 tbsp. pork panko
- 3 slices crispy bacon

Directions:

1. Warm up your mini Chaffle maker.
2. Combine the eggs, pork panko, and collagen peptides. Mix well. Divide the batter in two small bowls.

3. Once done, evenly distribute 1/2 of the crispy chopped bacon on the Chaffle maker.
4. Pour one bowl of the batter over the bacon. Cooking for 5 minutes and immediately repeat this step for the second chaffle.
5. Plate your cooked chaffles and sprinkle with extra Panko for an added crunch.
6. Enjoy!

Nutrition:

Calories: 266

Fats: 1g

Carbs: 11.2 g

Protein: 27 g

11. Chicken and Bacon Chaffles

Preparation Time: 5 minutes	Cooking Time: 8 minutes	Servings: 2

Ingredients:

- 1 organic egg, beaten
- 1/3 cup grass-fed cooked chicken, chopped
- 1 cooked bacon slice, crumbled
- 1/3 cup Pepper Jack cheese, shredded
- 1 teaspoon powdered ranch dressing

Directions:

1. Preheat a mini Chaffle iron and then grease it.
2. In a medium bowl, merge all ingredients and with a fork, mix until well blend.
3. Set half of the mixture into preheated Chaffle iron and Cooking for about 4 minutes or until golden brown.
4. Repeat with the remaining mixture.
5. Serve warm.

Nutrition:

Calories: 145

Fat: 9.4g

Carbohydrates: 1g

Sugar: 0.2g

Protein: 14.3g

12. Chaffle Katsu Sandwich

Preparation Time: 5 minutes

Cooking Time: 20 minutes

Servings: 4

Ingredients:

- For the chicken:
- 1/4 lb. boneless chicken thigh
- 1/8 tsp. salt
- 1/8 tsp. black pepper
- 1/2 cup almond flour
- 1 egg
- 3 oz. unflavored pork rinds
- 2 cup vegetable oil for deep frying For the brine:
- 2 cup of water
- 1 Tbsp. salt

For the sauce:

- 2 Tbsp. sugar-free ketchup
- 11/2 Tbsp. Worcestershire Sauce
- 1 Tbsp. oyster sauce
- 1 tsp. swerve/monk fruit For the chaffle:
- 2 egg
- 1 cup shredded mozzarella cheese

Directions:

1. Add brine ingredients in a large mixing bowl.
2. Add chicken and brine for 1 hour.

3. Pat chicken dry with a paper towel. Sprinkle with salt and pepper. Set aside.
4. Mix ketchup, oyster sauce, Worcestershire sauce, and swerve in a small mixing bowl.
5. Pulse pork rinds in a food processor, making fine crumbs.
6. Fill one bowl with flour, a second bowl with beaten eggs, and a third with crushed pork rinds.
7. Dip and coat each thigh in: flour, eggs, crushed pork rinds. Transfer on holding a plate.
8. Add oil to cover 1/2 inch of frying pan. Heat to 375F.
9. Once oil is hot, set heat to medium and add chicken. Cooking time depends on the chicken thickness.
10. Transfer to a drying rack.
11. Turn on Chaffle maker to heat and oil it with Cooking spray.
12. Beat egg in a small bowl.
13. Place 1/8 cup of cheese on Chaffle maker, then add1/4 of the egg mixture and top with 1/8 cup of cheese.
14. Cooking for 3-4 minutes.
15. Repeat for remaining batter.
16. Top chaffles with chicken katsu, 1 Tbsp. sauce, and another piece of chaffle.

Nutrition:

Carbs: 12 g

Fat: 1 g

Protein: 2 g

Calories: 57

13. Pork Rind Chaffles

Preparation Time: 5 minutes

Cooking Time: 10 minutes

Servings: 2

Ingredients:

- 1 organic egg, beaten
- 1/2 cup ground pork rinds
- 1/3 cup Mozzarella cheese, shredded
- Pinch of salt

Directions:

1. Preheat a mini Chaffle iron and then grease it.
2. In a bowl, set all the ingredients and beat until well blend.
3. Set half of the mixture into preheated Chaffle iron and Cooking for about 5 minutes or until golden brown.
4. Repeat with the remaining mixture.
5. Serve warm.

Nutrition:

Calories: 91

Fat: 5.9g

Carbohydrates: 0.3g

Sugar: 0.2g

Protein: 9.2g

Chapter 9. Dinner

14. Simple Blueberry Chaffle

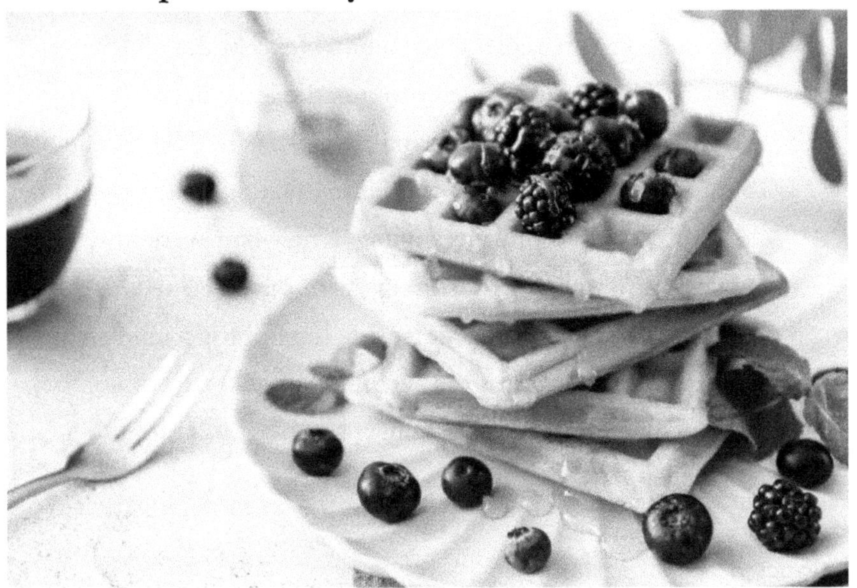

Preparation Time: 7 minutes

Cooking Time: 3 minutes

Servings: 2

Ingredients:

- 1 Egg (beaten)
- 1/2 cup of Mozzarella cheese (grated)
- 1 tsp. Erythritol
- 1/2 tsp. Baking powder
- 1 tsp. Blueberry extract
- 1/2 tsp. Cinnamon
- 12 Blueberries (fresh)

Directions:

1. Heat the mini-Chaffle maker with Cooking spray before ready to use.
2. Mix the entire ingredient*s in a bowl (except the blueberries). You should also use a mixer to mix the ingredients.
3. Pour ample batter into the Chaffle maker's middle and fan it out to the corners. If you overfill the first one, fill it up a little less every time to prevent spilling. 6 new blueberries on top
4. Allow 3 1/2 minutes to Cooking with the lid closed.
5. Remove the chaffle and set it aside to cool for 5 minutes on a cooling rack; repeat for the second chaffle. Add a dollop of whipped cream and a couple new blueberries on top.

Nutrition:

Calories: 121

Carbohydrates: 3g

Protein: 9g

Fat: 8g

Cholesterol: 104mg

Sodium: 208mg

15. Sweet Keto Chaffles

Preparation Time: 7 minutes

Cooking Time: 10 minutes

Servings: 2

Ingredients:

- 1 large egg
- 1/2 cup of shredded low moisture mozzarella
- 1/4 cup of almond flour
- 1/8 tsp. of gluten-free baking powder
- 3 tbsp. of granulated low-carb sweetener such as Erythritol or Swerve or brown sugar substitute

Directions:

1. To make the Chaffles, measure out all of the ingredients. Using a standard Chaffle maker to preheat a mini Chaffle maker.
2. You may either mix all of the ingredients together in a bowl or blend them together. In a mixer or food processor, mix the egg, mozzarella, almond flour, and baking powder.
3. After that, stir in the sweetener. The dough would be a bit runnier if the sweetener is added before mixing, so I like to add mine after.
4. Spoon one-third of the batter (3 to 4 tsp., around 55 g/1.9 oz.) into the hot Chaffle maker to produce three tiny Chaffles.
5. Cooking for 3 to 4 minutes with the Chaffle maker closed.

6. When you're done, remove the lid and set it aside to cool for a few moments. Transfer the chaffle to a cooling rack softly with a spatula. Continue for the remaining hitter.
7. Allow the chaffles to cool fully before serving. When they're hot, they'll be fluffy, but when they cool, they'll crisp up. Top with full-fat milk, coconut yogurt, whipped cream, bananas, and/or bacon syrup for a low-carb dessert. Serve with One-Minute Chocolate Milk, hot or cold!
8. Enjoy right away, or keep the chaffles in a sealed jar at room temperature for up to 3 days, or in the fridge for up to a week, without any toppings. The jar will hold them fluffy, but if you like them crispy, you can leave them out.

Nutrition:

Protein: 45

Fat: 47

Carbohydrates: 8

16. Easy Keto Sandwich Bowl

Preparation Time: 10 minutes

Cooking Time: 0 minutes

Servings: 1

Ingredients:

- 5 slices smoked deli ham
- 1 cup of chopped romaine hearts
- 3 slices provolone cheese
- 3 pickles
- 4 banana peppers
- 1/2 cucumber
- 1/3 orange bell pepper
- 3 cherry tomatoes

Dressing:

- 2 tbsp. olive oil
- 4 tsp. red wine vinegar
- 1/4 tsp. Italian seasoning

Directions:

1. Place the ham, cheese, and vegetables in a bowl and chop them up.
2. Mix together the olive oil, red wine vinegar, and Italian seasoning.
3. Toss the keto sandwich bowl with some dressing.

4. Have fun! (To allow the oil/vinegar mixture to infuse all of the other ingredients, let the keto sandwich bowl sit for a few minutes.)

Nutrition

Calories: 1037

Carbohydrates: 14g

Protein: 62g

Fat: 80g

Cholesterol: 162mg

Sodium: 4458mg

Potassium: 1393mg

17. Open-Faced Grilled Ham and Cheese Sandwich

Preparation Time: 10 minutes

Cooking Time: 15 minutes

Servings: 1

Ingredients:

- Olive oil
- 4 slices white toasted sandwich bread
- 1 tbsp. mustard
- 4 slices Applegate Naturals Slow cooked Ham
- 4 slices Applegate Organics American Cheese
- 2 thickly sliced tomatoes
- 1 thinly sliced red onion
- Salt and freshly ground black pepper
- Finely chopped chives, for garnish

Directions:

1. Heat the oven to 400F. Using olive oil, coat a small sheet pan.
2. Arrange the toast slices on the plate. Cover every slice of toast with 1 slice of ham, 1 slice of cheese, 2 slices of tomato, and a few slices of red onion, and spread the mustard on top.
3. Drizzle olive oil over every sandwich and season lightly with salt and pepper.
4. Bake for 10-12 minutes, or until the cheese is bubbling and melted. Serve immediately with chives as a garnish.

18. Cheesy Chaffle Sandwiches with Avocado and Bacon

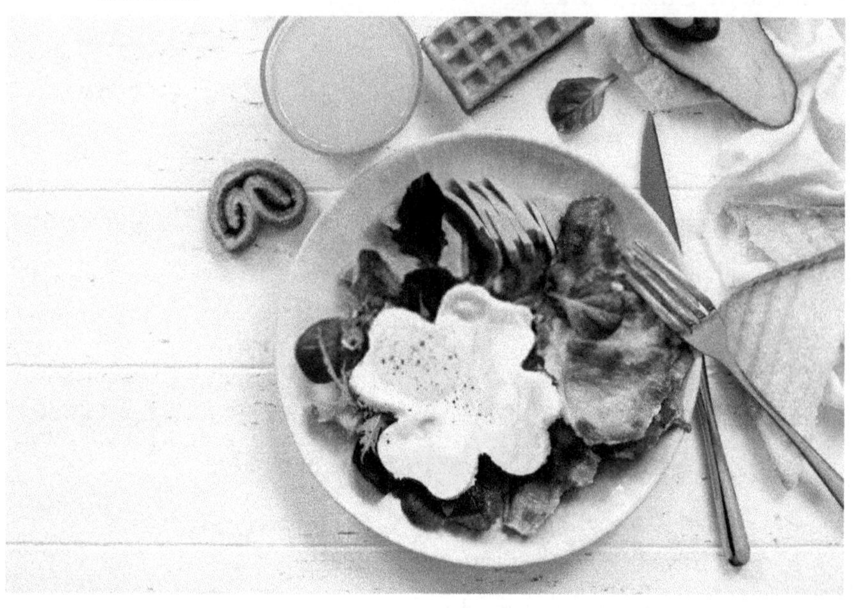

Preparation Time: 10 minutes

Cooking Time: 25 minutes

Servings: 8

Ingredients:

- 10 large eggs
- 11/4 cups of shredded sharp Cheddar cheese
- 2 slices center-cut bacon, cooked and crumbled
- 1/2 tsp. ground pepper
- 2 small sliced avocados
- 2 small sliced tomatoes
- 4 large leaves butter head lettuce

Directions:

1. In a bowl, whisk the egg*s until creamy. Add the cheese, crumbled bacon, and pepper as need.
2. Cover a 7-inch round Chaffle iron (not Belgian) with Cooking spray and preheat it. 2/3 cup of the egg mixture should be poured onto the molten Chaffle iron. Cooking for 4 to 5 minutes, or until the eggs are set and light golden brown. Go on for the remainder of the egg mixture and Cooking oil in the same manner (making 4 chaffles total).
3. Every chaffle should be quartered. Half of the quarters can be covered in avocado slices, tomato slices, and lettuce slices. Add the remaining chaffle quarters on to. Serve right away.

Nutrition:

Carbs 8 g

Fat 11 g

Protein 5 g

Calories 168

Chapter 10. Simple Chaffle

19. Broccoli Slaw with Pecans

Preparation time: 9 minutes

Cooking Time: 28 Minutes

Servings: 4

Ingredients:

- 2 tbsp. olive oil
- 2 cups broccoli slaw
- 1 red bell pepper, sliced
- 1 red onion, thinly sliced
- 1/2 cup toasted pecans, chopped
- 2 tbsp. flax seeds
- 1 tbsp. red wine vinegar
- 1/2 lemon, juiced
- 1 tsp. Dijon mustard
- 2 tbsp. mayonnaise
- 2 tbsp. chopped cilantro
- Salt and black pepper to taste

Directions:

1. In a bowl, thoroughly combine broccoli slaw, bell pepper, red onion, cilantro, salt, and pepper. Mix in pecans and flax seeds. In another small bowl, whisk the red wine vinegar, olive oil, lemon juice, mayonnaise, and mustard.
2. Drizzle the dressing over the slaw and serve.

20. Tomato Pizza with Strawberries

Preparation time: 9 minutes

Cooking Time: 40 Minutes

Servings: 4

Ingredients:

- 3 cups shredded mozzarella
- 2 tbsp. cream cheese, softened
- 3/4 cup almond flour
- 2 tbsp. almond meal 1 celery stalk, chopped
- 1 tomato, chopped
- 1 tbsp. olive oil
- 2 tbsp. balsamic vinegar
- 1 cup strawberries, halved
- 1 tbsp. chopped mint leaves

Directions:

1. Preheat oven to 390 F. Line a pizza pan with parchment paper. Microwave 2 cups of mozzarella cheese and cream cheese for 1 minute.
2. Remove and mix in almond flour and almond meal. Spread the mixture on the pizza pan and bake for 10 minutes. Spread remaining mozzarella cheese on the crust. In a bowl, toss celery, tomato, olive oil, and balsamic vinegar. Spoon the mixture onto the mozzarella cheese and arrange the strawberries on top.
3. Top with mint leaves. Bake for 15 minutes. Serve sliced.

Nutrition:

Cal 306

Net Carbs 4g

Fats 11g

Protein 28g

21. Broccoli “Rice” with Walnuts

Preparation time: 15 minutes	Cooking Time: 25 Minutes	Servings: 4

Ingredients:

- 2 heads large broccoli, riced
- 2 tbsp. butter
- 1 garlic clove, minced
- 1/4 cup toasted walnuts, chopped
- 4 tbsp. sesame seeds, toasted
- 1/2 cup vegetable broth
- 2 tbsp. chopped cilantro
- Salt and black pepper to taste

Directions:

1. Melt butter in a pot and stir in garlic. Cooking until fragrant, for 1 minute and add in broccoli and vegetable broth. Allow steaming for 2 minutes.
2. Season with salt and pepper and Cooking for 3-5 minutes. Pour in walnuts, sesame seeds, and cilantro. Fluff the rice and serve warm.

Nutrition:

Cal 239

Net Carbs 3g

Fat 15g

Protein 9g

Chapter 11. Sweets

22. Chocolate Chip Chaffles

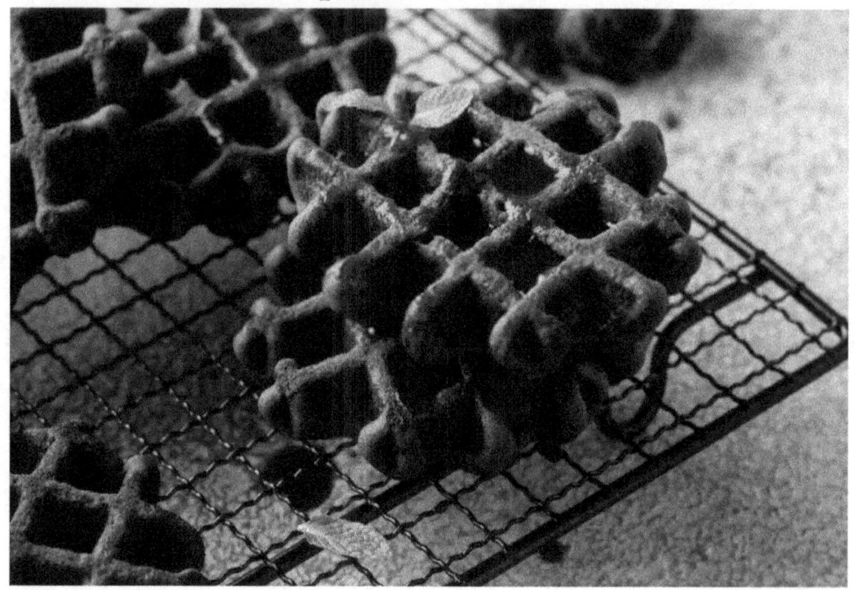

Preparation Time: 3 minutes

Cooking Time: 8 minutes

Serving: 2

Ingredients:

- 1/2 cup grated mozzarella cheese
- 1/2 tbsp. granulated Swerve, or sweetener of choice
- 1 tbsp. almond flour, ALLERGY WARNING
- 2 tbsp. low carb, sugar-free chocolate chips
- 1 egg
- 1/4 tsp. cinnamon

Directions:

1. Preheat your Chaffle iron.
2. In a bowl, merge the almond flour, egg, cinnamon, mozzarella cheese, Swerve, chocolate chips.
3. Place half the batter in the Chaffle iron and Cooking for four minutes.
4. Remove chaffle and Cooking the remaining batter.
5. Let chaffles cool before serving.

Nutrition

Calories: 136 kcal

Cholesterol: 104 mg

Carbohydrates: 2 g

Protein: 10 g

Fat: 10 g

Sugar: 1 g

23. Chocolate Chaffle Recipe

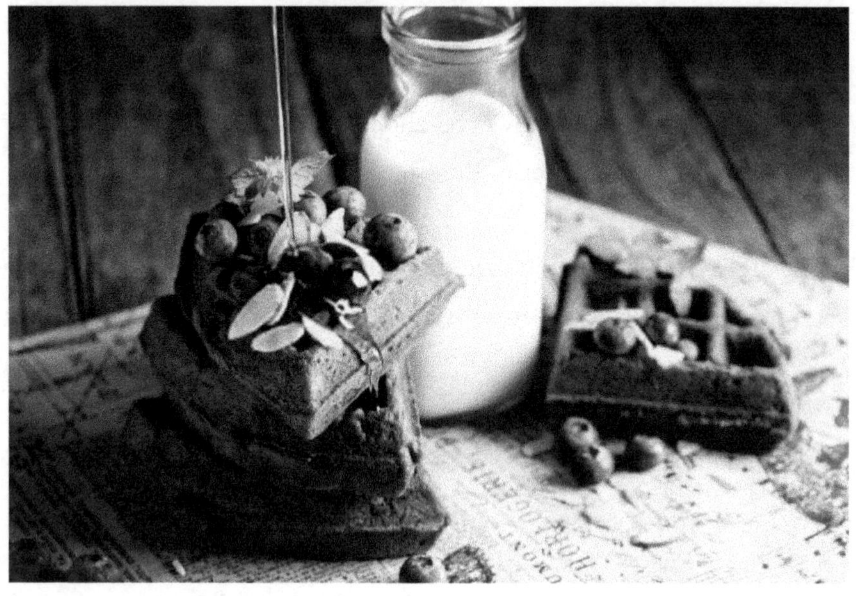

Preparation Time: 3 minutes

Cooking Time: 8 minutes

Serving: 2

Ingredients:

- 1 tsp. vanilla extract
- 1 tbsp. cocoa powder, unsweetened.
- 1 egg
- 2 tbsp. almond flour, ALLERGY WARNING
- 2 tsp. monk fruit
- 1 oz. cream cheese

Directions:

1. Preheat the Chaffle iron.

2. Soften the cream cheese then whisk together the other ingredients well.
3. Set the batter into the center of the Chaffle iron and spread out.
4. Cooking batter for between three and five minutes.
5. Remove chaffle once set and serve.

Nutrition

Calories: 261 kcal

Carbohydrates: 4 g net

Protein: 11.5 g

Fat: 22.2 g

24. S'mores Chaffles

Preparation Time: 30 minutes

Cooking Time: 20 minutes

Serving: 2

Ingredients:

Chaffle Ingredients:

- 1 egg
- 1/2 tsp. vanilla extract
- 1/4 cup cream cheese
- 2 tbsp. almond flour, ALLERGY WARNING
- 1 tbsp. sweetener of choice
- 1 tbsp. protein powder, unflavored
- 1/2 tsp. baking powder
- 1 tsp. ground cinnamon

For Sugar-Free Marshmallow:

- 100 g (3.5 oz.,) xylitol, or other baking friendly sweetener
- 3 tbsp. water
- 4 gelatin sheets, or 7 g gelatin powder

For Chocolate Dip:

- 10 g cacao butter
- 80 g sugar-free chocolate

Directions for Sugar-Free Marshmallow:

1. If you do not have sugar-free marshmallow fluff, then it is suggested that you make this up to eight hours, or even the day before, making the chaffle.
2. Choose a container to set the marshmallow in later. This container needs to be lined with cling film.
3. Gelatin sheets need to be placed in water for a few minutes before use.
4. Melt the sugar in a Cooking pot and allow boiling for up to three minutes before adding the gelatin sheets or powder.
5. Dissolve the gelatin fully.
6. Now that the liquid is ready, pour it into an electric mixer.
7. Mix the mixture until the liquid bulks up and starts to form a white marshmallow-like fluff.
8. Pour the marshmallow fluff into the previously prepared container and smooth the surface.
9. Allow the mixture to sit on a kitchen surface for no less than eight hours. For the best possible setting, allow for the fluff to rest overnight to allow it to set into the marshmallow form. Cover with cling film once cool to prevent insects from getting into the mixture.
10. Once fully set, the marshmallow can be cut into the desired shape.
11. Dust the marshmallow pieces with powdered sweetener if you want to keep it softer for longer.

Chaffle Directions:

1. Preheat the Chaffle iron.
2. Beat the egg before adding the cinnamon.

3. Combine the remaining chaffle ingredients before adding a few drops of vanilla.
4. Divide the batter in half and Cooking each portion for three minutes.
5. Set chaffles aside to cool.
6. If you want to prepare the s'mores at home, take the marshmallow fluff and spread it to the thickness of choice on one chaffle before adding the second chaffle on top.
7. Set aside the chaffles to prepare the chocolate dip.

Directions for Chocolate Dip:

1. Make use of a double boiler or instant pot to melt the cocoa butter and sugar-free chocolate together.
2. Make sure the mixture is completely smooth before dipping the chaffle's edges in it. Coat all the marshmallow fluff.
3. Put aside and allow the chocolate to harden.

Nutrition

Calories: 368 kcal

Carbohydrates: 3 g

Protein: 11 g

Fat: 23 g

25. Thin Mint Cookies Chaffles

Preparation Time: 20 minutes

Cooking Time: 16 minutes

Serving: 4

Ingredients:

Chaffle Ingredients:

- 1 cup grated mozzarella cheese
- 2 tbsp. unsweetened cocoa powder
- 2 large eggs
- 3 tbsp. Swerve confectioners, or sweetener of choice

For Filling:

- 6 oz. cream cheese, softened
- 2 tbsp. unsweetened cocoa powder
- 1/2 cup almond flour
- 1/4 cup Swerve confectioners, or sweeteners of choice
- 1 tsp. peppermint extract
- 1/2 tsp. vanilla extract

For Topping:

- 3 tbsp. sugar-free chocolate chips
- 1 tbsp. coconut oil, ALLERGY WARNING

Directions:

For Chaffle

1. Preheat the Chaffle iron.

2. Mix all the chaffle ingredients in a bowl and make sure everything is mixed well.
3. Cooking 1/4 of the batter in the Chaffle iron for two to four minutes. The longer it is cooked, the crispier it becomes.
4. Continue to make chaffles until the batter is finished.

Directions

For Filling and Topping:

1. Combine all the filler ingredients and beat with a hand mixer on high.
2. Apply the filling to the three cooled chaffles, stack, and set aside.
3. Heat the coconut oil and chocolate chips at 30-second intervals in a microwave until melted together.
4. Drizzle this over the stacked chaffles and serve.

Nutrition

Calories: 431 kcal

Carbohydrates: 6 g net

Protein: 16 g

Fat: 38 g

26. Strawberry Chaffle

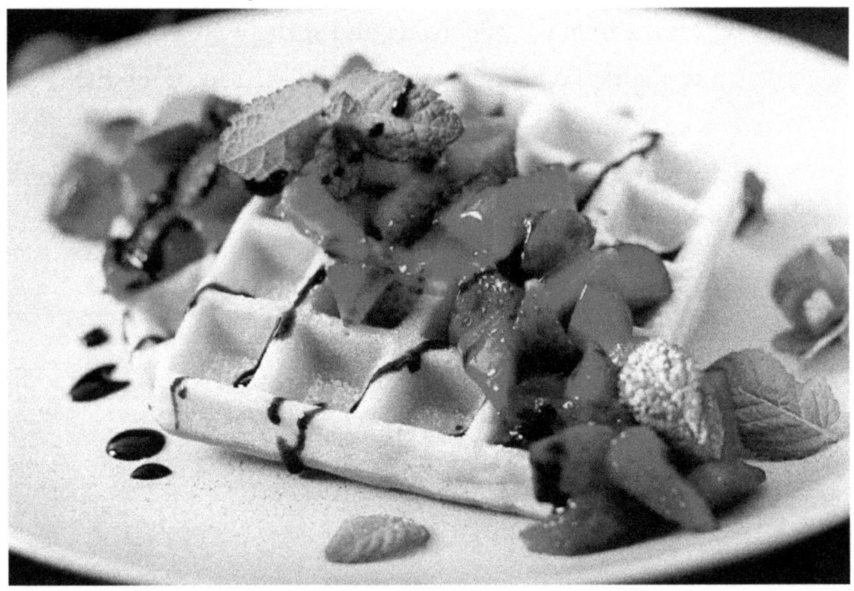

Preparation Time: 20 minutes

Cooking Time: 16 minutes

Serving: 2

Ingredients:

- Sliced strawberries (2 fresh)
- Egg (1)
- Vanilla (1 tsp.)
- Baking powder (.25 tsp.)
- Shredded mozzarella cheese (.25 cup)
- Cream cheese (1 tbsp.)

Directions:

1. Preheat the mini Chaffle maker and spritz with a bit of Cooking spray. Whisk the egg and add the rest of the fixings to make the batter.
2. Prepare the batter in two batches, Cooking them until golden or about four minutes.

Nutrition:

Calories 210

Total Fat 17 g

Saturated Fat 10 g

Cholesterol 110 mg

Sodium 250 mg

Chapter 12. Savory

27. Avocado Chaffle

Preparation Time: 5 minutes | Cooking Time: 10 minutes | Servings: 2

Ingredients

- 1/2 avocado, sliced
- 1/2 tsp. lemon juice
- 1/8 tsp. salt
- 1/8 tsp. black pepper
- 1 egg
- 1/2 cup shredded cheese
- 1/4 crumbled feta cheese
- 1 cherry tomato, halved

Directions:

1. Merge together avocado, lemon juice, salt, and pepper until well-combined.
2. Turn on Chaffle maker to heat and oil it with Cooking spray.
3. Beat egg in a small mixing bowl.
4. Place 1/8 cup of cheese on Chaffle maker, then spread half of the egg mixture over it and top with 1/8 cup of cheese.
5. Close and Cooking for 3-4 minutes. Repeat for remaining batter.
6. Let chaffles cool for 3-4 minutes, and then spread avocado mix on top of each.
7. Top with crumbled feta and cherry tomato halves.

28. Zucchini and Onion Chaffles

Preparation Time: 5 minutes

Cooking Time: 16 minutes

Servings: 4

Ingredients

- 2 cups zucchini, grated and squeezed
- 1/2 cup onion, grated and squeezed
- 2 organic eggs
- 1/2 cup Mozzarella cheese, shredded
- 1/2 cup Parmesan cheese, grated

Directions:

1. Preheat a Chaffle iron and then grease it.
2. In a medium bowl, set all ingredients and, mix until well combined.
3. Place 1/4 of the mixture into preheated Chaffle iron and Cooking for about 4 minutes or until golden brown.
4. Repeat with the remaining mixture.
5. Serve warm.

29. Jalapeño Chaffles

Preparation Time: 5 minutes

Cooking Time: 10 minutes

Servings: 2

Ingredients

- 1 organic egg, beaten
- 1/2 cup Cheddar cheese, shredded
- 1/2 tablespoon jalapeño pepper, chopped
- Salt, to taste

Directions:

1. Preheat a mini Chaffle iron and then grease it.
2. In a medium bowl, set all ingredients and with a fork, mix until well combined.
3. Set half of the mixture into preheated Chaffle iron and Cooking for about 5 minutes or until golden brown.
4. Repeat with the remaining mixture.
5. Serve warm.

30. Three-cheeses Herbed Chaffles

Preparation Time: 5 minutes

Cooking Time: 12 minutes

Servings: 4

Ingredients

- 4 tablespoons almond flour
- 1 tablespoon coconut flour
- 1 teaspoon mixed dried herbs
- 1/2 teaspoon organic baking powder
- 1/4 teaspoon garlic powder
- 1/4 teaspoon onion powder
- Salt and freshly ground black pepper
- 1/4 cup cream cheese, softened
- 3 large organic eggs
- 1/2 cup Cheddar cheese, grated
- 1/3 cup Parmesan cheese, grated

Directions:

1. Preheat a Chaffle iron and then grease it.
2. In a bowl, mix together the flours, dried herbs, baking powder and seasoning and mix well.
3. In a separate bowl, merge cream cheese and eggs and beat until well combined.
4. Add the flour mixture, cheddar and Parmesan cheese and mix until well combined.

5. Place the desired amount of the mixture into preheated Chaffle iron and Cooking for about 2-3 minutes or until golden brown.
6. Repeat with the remaining mixture.
7. Serve warm.

Nutrition:

Calories: 240

Net Carb: 2.6g

Fat: 19gSaturated

Fat: 5g

Carbohydrates: 4g

Dietary Fiber: 1.6g

Sugar: 0.7g

Protein: 12.3g

31. Bagel Seasoning Chaffles

Preparation Time: 15 minutes

Cooking Time: 20 minutes

Servings: 4

Ingredients

- 1 large organic egg
- 1 cup Mozzarella cheese, shredded
- 1 tablespoon almond flour
- 1 teaspoon organic baking powder
- 2 teaspoons bagel seasoning
- 1/4 teaspoon garlic powder
- 1/4 teaspoon onion powder

Directions:

1. Preheat a mini Chaffle iron and then grease it.
2. In a medium bowl, set all ingredients and with a fork, mix until well combined.
3. Place 1/4 of the mixture into preheated Chaffle iron and Cooking for about 4 minutes or until golden brown.
4. Repeat with the remaining mixture.
5. Serve warm.

Nutrition:

Calories: 73

Net Carb: 2g

Fat: 5.5g

Saturated Fat: 1.5g

Carbohydrates: 2.3g

Dietary Fiber: 0.3g

Sugar: 0.9g

Protein: 3.7g

Chapter 13. Festive

32. Swiss Bacon chaffle

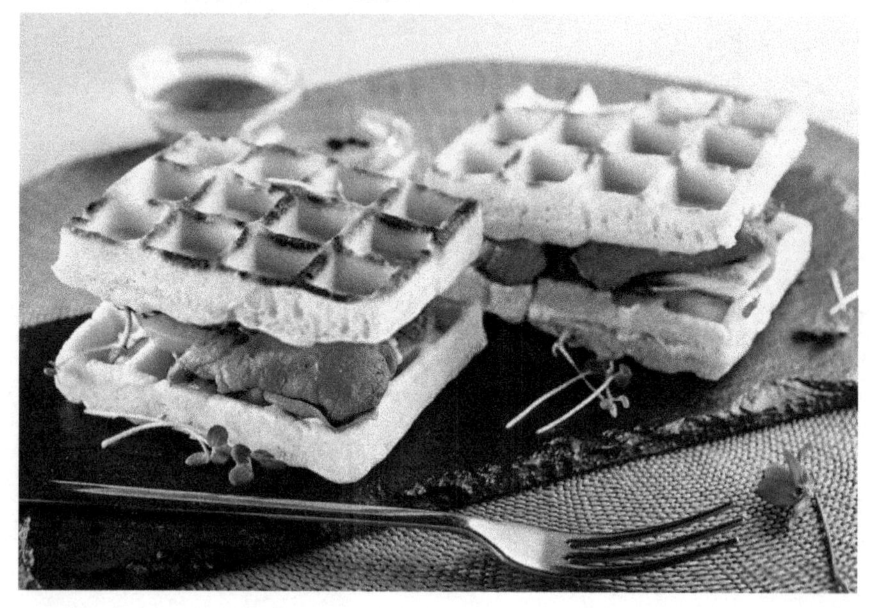

Preparation time: 10 minutes

Cooking Time: 8 Minutes

Servings: 2

Ingredients:

- 1 egg
- 1/2 cup Swiss cheese
- 2 tablespoons Cooked crumbled bacon

Directions:

1. Preheat your Chaffle maker.
2. Beat the egg in a bowl.
3. Stir in the cheese and bacon.

4. Pour half of the mixture into the device.
5. Close and Cook for 4 minutes.
6. Cook the second chaffle using the same steps.

Nutrition

Calories 23

Total Fat 17.6g

Saturated Fat 8.1g

Cholesterol 128mg

Sodium 522mg

Total Carbohydrate 1.9g

Dietary Fiber 0g

Total Sugars 0.5g

Protein 17.1g

Potassium 158mg

33. Chili Taco Chaffle

Preparation time: 8 minutes

Cooking Time: 20 Minutes

Servings: 2

Ingredients:

- 1 tablespoon olive oil
- 1 lb. ground beef
- 1 teaspoon ground cumin
- 1 teaspoon chili powder
- 1/4 teaspoon onion powder
- 1/2 teaspoon garlic powder
- Salt to taste
- 4 basic chaffles
- 1 cup cabbage, chopped
- 4 tablespoons salsa (sugar-free)

Directions:

1. Pour the olive oil into a pan over medium heat.
2. Add the ground beef.
3. Season with the salt and spices.
4. Cooking until brown and crumbly.
5. Fold the chaffle to create a "taco shell".
6. Stuff each chaffle taco with cabbage.
7. Top with the ground beef and salsa.

Nutrition

Calories 255

Total Fat 10.9g

Saturated Fat 3.2g

Cholesterol 101mg

Sodium 220mg

Potassium 561mg

Total Carbohydrate 3g

Dietary Fiber 1g

Protein 35.1g

Total Sugars 1.3g

34. Keto Coffee Chaffles

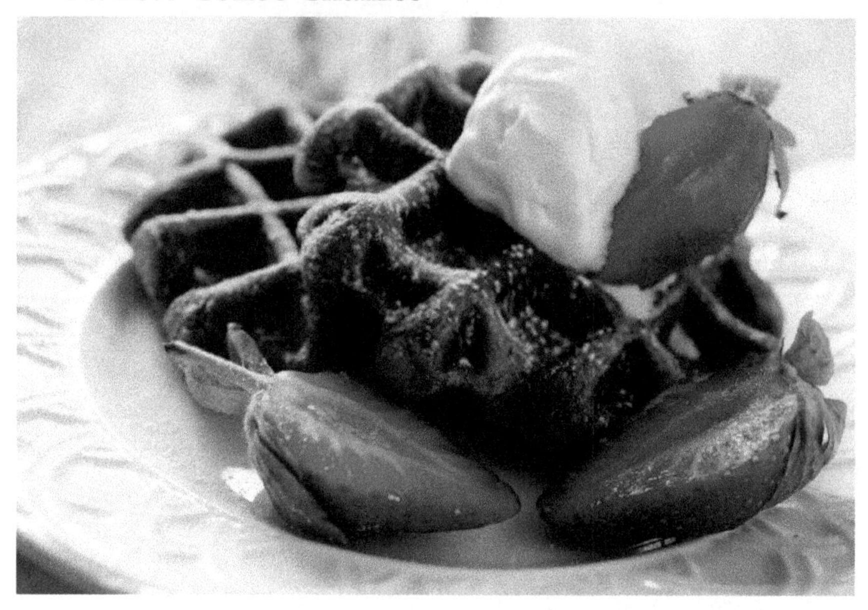

Preparation Time: 7 minutes

Cooking Time: 5 minutes

Servings: 2

Ingredients:

- 1 tbsp. almond flour
- 1 tbsp. instant coffee
- 1/2 cup cheddar cheese
- 1/2 tsp. baking powder
- 1 large egg

Directions:

1. Warmth Chaffle iron and grease with Cooking spray

2. Meanwhile, in a small mixing bowl, mix together all ingredients and 1/2 cup cheese.
3. Pour 1/8 cup cheese in a Chaffle maker and then pour the mixture in the center of greased Chaffle.
4. Again, sprinkle cheese on the batter.
5. Close the Chaffle maker.
6. Cooking chaffles for about 4-5 minutes until Cooked and crispy.
7. Once chaffles are cooked, remove and enjoy!

Nutrition

Protein: 26

Fat: 69

Carbohydrates: 5

35. Crunchy Chaffle Cake

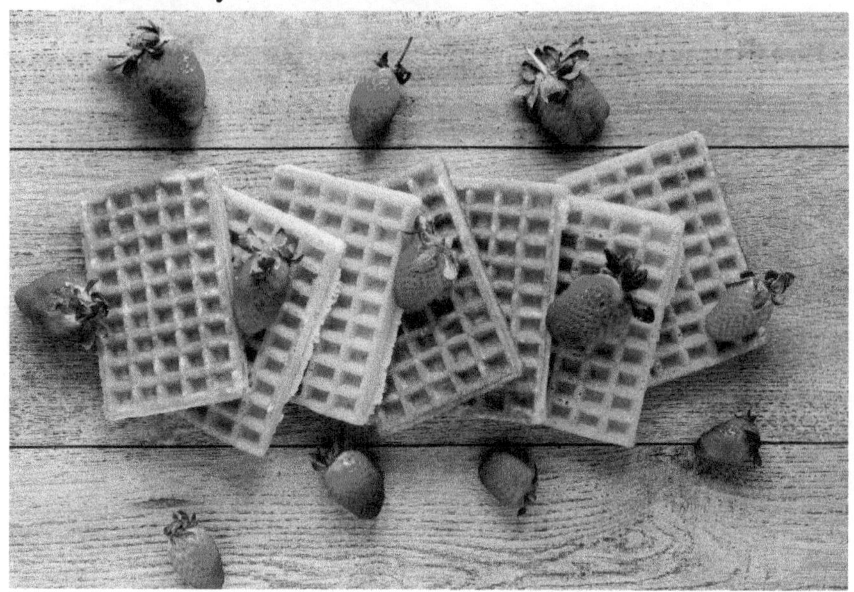

Preparation time: 2 minutes

Cooking time: 8 minutes

Servings 2

Ingredients:

- 1 egg
- 2 tablespoons almond flour
- 1/2 teaspoon coconut flour
- 20 drops Captain Cereal flavoring
- 1 tablespoon cream cheese
- 1/4 teaspoon baking powder
- 1/4 teaspoon vanilla extract
- 1/8 teaspoon xanthan gum
- 1 tablespoon butter, melted

- 1 tablespoon Swerve

Directions

1. Preheat the mini Chaffle maker.
2. Whisk all the ingredients until smooth and creamy in a large bowl. Allow the batter to rest for a few minutes.
3. Add about 2 to 3 tablespoons of batter to your Chaffle maker and cook for about 3 minutes. Repeat with remaining batter.
4. Serve immediately.

36. Jicama Chaffle

Preparation time: 2 minutes

Cooking time: 8 minutes

Servings 4

- Ingredients:
- 1 large jicama root, peeled, shredded
- 2 eggs, whisked
- 1 cup shredded Cheddar cheese
- 1/2 medium onion, minced
- 2 garlic cloves, pressed
- Salt and ground black pepper, to taste

Directions:

1. Preheat the Chaffle maker.
2. Place shredded jicama in a large colander, sprinkle with salt. Mix well and allow draining. Squeeze out as much liquid as possible.
3. Microwave the salted jicama for 5 to 8 minutes.
4. Combine the jicama with the remaining ingredients in a large bowl.
5. Sprinkle a little more cheese on Chaffle maker before adding 3 tablespoons of the mixture, sprinkle a little more cheese on top of the mixture
6. Cook for 5 minutes. Flip and cook 2 minutes more.
7. Serve immediately.

Nutrition:

Calories: 168

Fat: 11.8g

Protein: 10.0g

Carbs: 5.1g

Net Carbs: 3.4g

Fiber: 1.7g

Chapter 14. Vegetarian

37. Cauliflower Chaffle

Preparation Time: 5 minutes

Cooking Time: 15 minutes

Serving: 4

Ingredients:

Batter

- 4 eggs
- 2 cups grated cheddar cheese
- 1 cup steamed cauliflower, chopped
- Salt and pepper to taste
- 1 teaspoon dried basil
- 1/2 teaspoon onion powder
- 2 tablespoons almond flour
- 2 teaspoons baking powder

Other

- 2 tablespoons Cooking spray to brush the Chaffle maker
- 1/4 cup mascarpone cheese for serving

Directions

1. Preheat the Chaffle maker.
2. Add the eggs, grated cheddar, cauliflower, salt and pepper, dried basil, onion powder, almond flour and baking powder to a bowl.
3. Mix with a fork.

4. Brush the heated Chaffle maker with Cooking spray and add a few tablespoons of the batter.
5. Close the lid and Cooking for about 5–7 minutes depending on your Chaffle maker.
6. Serve each chaffle with mascarpone cheese.

Nutrition

Calories 409

Fat 33.7 g,

Carbs 5 g

Sugar 1.4 g,

Protein 22.7 g

Sodium 434 Mg

38. Celery and Cottage Cheese Chaffle

Preparation Time: 5 minutes

Cooking Time: 15 minutes

Serving: 4

Ingredients:

Batter

- 4 eggs
- 2 cups grated cheddar cheese
- 1 cup fresh celery, chopped
- Salt and pepper to taste
- 2 tablespoons chopped almonds
- 2 teaspoons baking powder

Other

- 2 tablespoons Cooking spray to brush the Chaffle maker
- 1/4 cup cottage cheese for serving

Directions

1. Preheat the Chaffle maker.
2. Add the eggs, grated mozzarella cheese, chopped celery, salt and pepper, chopped almonds and baking powder to a bowl.
3. Mix with a fork.
4. Brush the heated Chaffle maker with Cooking spray and add a few tablespoons of the batter.
5. Close the lid and Cooking for about 5–7 minutes depending on your Chaffle maker.
6. Serve each chaffle with cottage cheese on top.

Nutrition

Calories 385

Fat 31.6 G

Carbs 4 G

Sugar 1.5 G,

Protein 22.2 G

Sodium 492 Mg

39. Zucchini in Chaffles

Preparation time: 10 minutes	Cooking Time: 18 Minutes	Servings: 2

Ingredients:

- 2 large zucchinis, grated and squeezed
- 2 large organic eggs
- 2/3 cup Cheddar cheese, shredded
- 2 tablespoons coconut flour
- 1/2 teaspoon garlic powder
- 1/2 teaspoon red pepper flakes, crushed
- Salt, to taste

Directions:

1. Preheat a Chaffle iron and then grease it.
2. In a medium bowl, set all ingredients and, mix until well combined.
3. Place 1/4 of the mixture into preheated Chaffle iron and Cooking for about 4-41/2 minutes or until golden brown.
4. Repeat with the remaining mixture.
5. Serve warm.

Nutrition:

Calories 311

Protein 16 g

Carbs 17 g

Fat 15 g

40. Oniony Pickled Chaffles

Preparation Time: 25 minutes

Cooking Time: 7 minutes

Serving: 2

Ingredients:

- Egg: 1
- Onion: 1/2 cup finely chopped
- Cheddar Cheese: 1/2 cup (shredded)
- Pork panko: 1/2 cup
- Pickle slices: 6-8 thin
- Pickle juice: 1 tbsp.

Direction:

1. Mix egg, onion, cheese, and pork panko
2. Fill in a thin layer on a preheated Chaffle iron
3. Remove any excess juice from pickles
4. Add pickle slices and pour again more mixture over the top
5. Cooking the chaffle for around 5 minutes
6. Make as many Chaffles as your mixture and Chaffle maker allow

Nutrition

Calories: 366

Fat: 27g

Protein: 10g

Chapter 15. Meat

41. BBQ Sauce Pork Chaffle

Preparation Time: 5 minutes

Cooking Time: 15 minutes

Serving: 4

Ingredients:

- 1/2 pound ground pork
- 3 eggs
- 1 cup grated mozzarella cheese
- Salt and pepper to taste
- 1 clove garlic, minced
- 1 teaspoon dried rosemary
- 3 tablespoons sugar-free BBQ sauce
- 2 tablespoons butter to brush the Chaffle maker
- 1/2 pound pork rinds for serving
- 1/4 cup sugar-free BBQ sauce for serving

Directions

1. Preheat the Chaffle maker.
2. Add the ground pork, eggs, mozzarella, salt and pepper, minced garlic, dried rosemary, and BBQ sauce to a bowl.
3. Mix until combined.
4. Brush the heated Chaffle maker with butter and add a few tablespoons of the batter.
5. Close the lid and Cooking for about 7–8 minutes depending on your Chaffle maker.

6. Serve each chaffle with some pork rinds and a tablespoon of BBQ sauce.

Nutrition

Calories 350

Fat 21.1 g

Carbs 2.7 g

Sugar 0.3 g,

Protein 36.9 g

Sodium 801 Mg

42. Rosemary Pork Chops on Chaffle

Preparation Time: 5 minutes

Cooking Time: 15 minutes

Serving: 4

Ingredients:

- 4 eggs
- 2 cups grated mozzarella cheese
- Salt and pepper to taste
- Pinch of nutmeg
- 2 tablespoons sour cream
- 6 tablespoons almond flour
- 2 teaspoons baking powder

Pork chops

- 2 tablespoons olive oil
- 1 pound pork chops
- Salt and pepper to taste
- 1 teaspoon freshly chopped rosemary

Other

- 2 tablespoons Cooking spray to brush the Chaffle maker
- 2 tablespoons freshly chopped basil for decoration

Directions

1. Preheat the Chaffle maker.
2. Add the eggs, mozzarella cheese, salt and pepper, nutmeg, sour cream, almond flour and baking powder to a bowl.

3. Mix until combined.
4. Brush the heated Chaffle maker with Cooking spray and add a few tablespoons of the batter.
5. Close the lid and Cooking for about 5-7 minutes depending on your Chaffle maker.
6. Meanwhile, heat the butter in a nonstick grill pan and season the pork chops with salt and pepper and freshly chopped rosemary.
7. Cooking the pork chops for about 4–5 minutes on each side.
8. Serve each chaffle with a pork chop and sprinkle some freshly chopped basil on top.

Nutrition

Calories 66

Fat 55.2 g

Carbs 4.8 g

Sugar 0.4 g,

Protein 37.5 g

Sodium 235 Mg

43. Savory Beef Chaffle

Preparation Time: 10 minutes

Cooking Time: 15 minutes

Servings: 2

Ingredients:

- 1 teaspoon olive oil
- 2 cups ground beef
- Garlic salt to taste
- 1 red bell pepper, sliced into strips
- 1 green bell pepper, sliced into strips
- 1 onion, minced
- 1 bay leaf
- 2 garlic chaffles
- Butter

Directions:

1. Put your pan over medium heat.
2. Add the olive oil and Cooking ground beef until brown.
3. Season with garlic salt and add bay leaf.
4. Drain the fat, transfer to a plate and set aside.
5. Discard the bay leaf.
6. In the same pan, Cooking the onion and bell peppers for 2 minutes.
7. Put the beef back to the pan.
8. Heat for 1 minute.
9. Spread butter on top of the chaffle.
10. Add the ground beef and veggies.

11. Roll or fold the chaffle.

Nutrition:

Calories 220   Total Fat 17.8g

Protein 27.1g

44. Mediterranean Lamb Kebabs on Chaffles

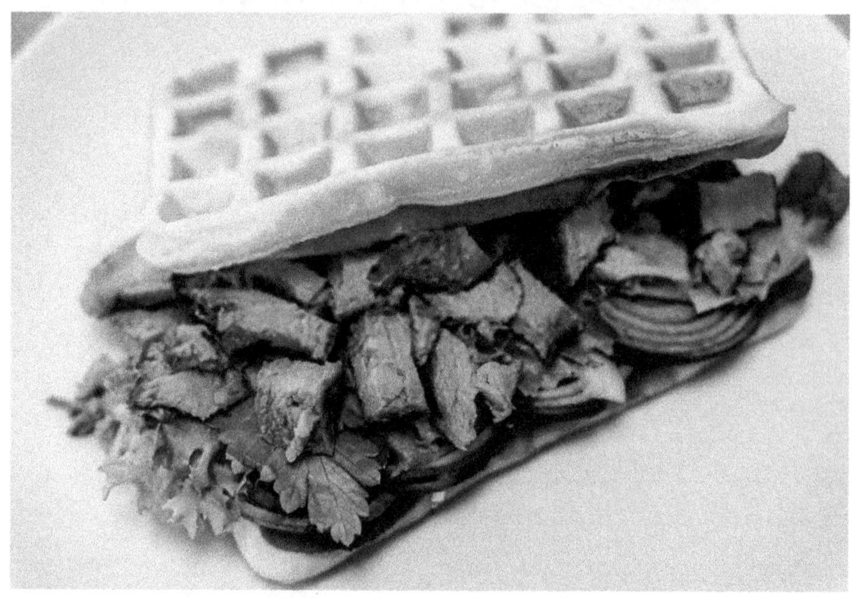

Preparation time: 10 minutes

Cooking Time: 15 Minutes

Servings: 2

Ingredients:

- 4 eggs
- 2 cups grated mozzarella cheese
- Salt and pepper to taste
- 1 teaspoon garlic powder
- 1/4 cup Greek yogurt
- 1/2 cup coconut flour
- 2 teaspoons baking powder
- 1 pound ground lamb meat
- Salt and pepper to taste

- 1 egg
- 2 tablespoons almond flour
- 1 spring onion, finely chopped
- 1/2 teaspoon dried garlic
- 2 tablespoons olive oil
- 2 tablespoons butter to brush the Chaffle maker
- 1/4 cup sour cream for serving
- 4 sprigs of fresh dill for garnish

Directions:

1. Preheat the Chaffle maker.
2. Add the eggs, mozzarella cheese, salt and pepper, garlic powder, Greek yogurt, coconut flour and baking powder to a bowl.
3. Mix until combined.
4. Brush the heated Chaffle maker with butter and add a few tablespoons of the batter.
5. Close the lid and Cooking for about 7 minutes depending on your Chaffle maker.
6. Meanwhile, add the ground lamb, salt and pepper, egg, almond flour, chopped spring onion, and dried garlic to a bowl. Mix and form medium-sized kebabs.
7. Impale each kebab on a skewer. Warmth the olive oil in a frying pan.
8. Cooking the lamb kebabs for about 3 minutes on each side.
9. Serve each chaffle with a tablespoon of sour cream and one or two lamb kebabs. Decorate with fresh dill.

Nutrition:

Calories 132

Protein 10 g

Fat 0 g

Cholesterol 0 mg

Potassium 353 mg

Calcium 9 mg

Fiber 1.9 g

Chapter 16. Cakes and Sandwiches

45. Strawberry Shortcake Chaffle

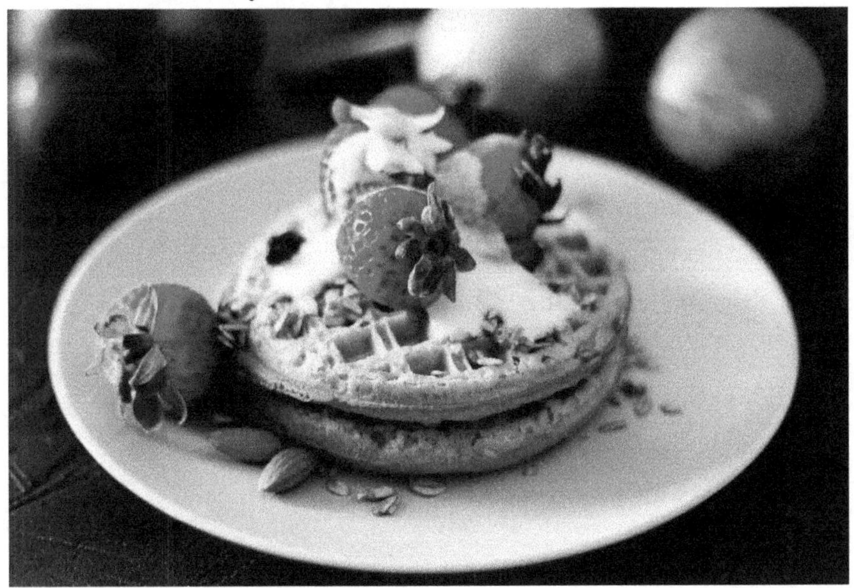

Preparation Time: 5 minutes

Cooking Time: 10 minutes

Servings: 2

Ingredients:

- Egg: 1
- Heavy Whipping Cream: 1 tbsp.
- Any non-sugar sweetener: 2 tbsp.
- Coconut Flour: 1 tsp.
- Cake batter extract: 1/2 tsp.
- Baking powder: 1/4 tsp.
- Strawberry: 4 or as per your taste

Directions:

1. Preheat a mini Chaffle maker if needed and grease it
2. In a mixing bowl, beat eggs and add non-sugar sweetener, coconut flour, baking powder, and cake batter extract
3. Merge them all well and pour the mixture to the lower plate of the Chaffle maker
4. Close the lid
5. Cooking for at least 4 minutes to get the desired crunch
6. Remove the chaffle from the heat and keep aside for around two minutes
7. Make as many chaffles as your mixture and Chaffle maker allow
8. Serve with whipped cream and strawberries on top

Nutrition:

Calories 334

Fat 12.1g

Protein 48.2g

46. Creamy Pumpkin Pie

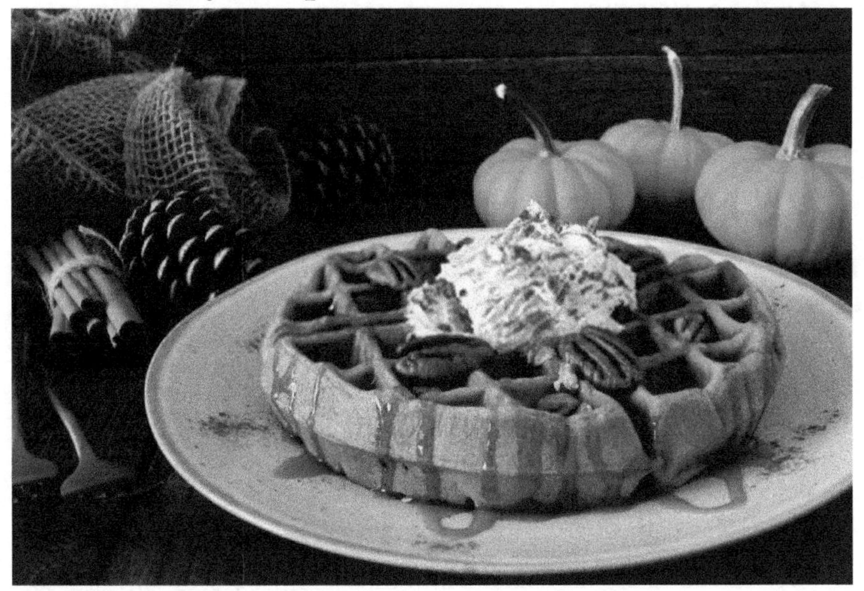

Preparation Time: 15 minutes

Cooking Time: 45 minutes

Servings: 6

Ingredients

For crust:

- 1 cup almond flour
- 2 tbsp. butter

For pie filling:

- 1 egg
- 1 tsp. vanilla
- 1/4 tsp. allspice
- 1/4 tsp. ground ginger

- 1/4 tsp. ground cloves
- 1 tsp. cinnamon
- 1 lemon zest
- 1/2 cup of coconut milk
- 1/2 swerve
- 1 cup pumpkin puree

Direction

1. Grease a 6-inch spring-form pan with butter and set aside.
2. Add all crust ingredients into the bowl and mix until combined.
3. Transfer crust mixture to the pan and spread evenly with the palm of your hands. Place in freezer for 15 minutes.
4. Add all filling ingredients into the food processor and process until smooth.
5. Pour filling mixture into the crust in spring-form pan.
6. Cover spring form pan with aluminum foil.
7. Pour 1 cup of water into the instant pot then place a trivet in the pot.
8. Place the pie spring-form pan on top of the trivet.
9. Seal pot with lid and select manual and set timer for 35 minutes.
10. Allow to release pressure naturally for 15 minutes then release using the quick release method.
11. Open the lid carefully. Remove pan from the pot and let it cool completely.
12. Place pie in refrigerator for 4 hours.
13. Serve chilled and enjoy.

Nutrition:

Calories 215

Fat 18.8 g

Carbohydrates 9.2 g

Sugar 2.8 g

Protein 5.9 g

Cholesterol 37 mg

47. Delicious Almond Peach Pie

Preparation Time: 10 minutes

Cooking Time: 15 minutes

Servings: 6

Ingredients

- 4 large eggs
- 1 tsp. lemon zest
- 1/2 tsp. vanilla
- 3 1/2 tbsp. swerve
- 1 1/2 tsp. baking powder
- 6 tbsp. butter
- 1/4 cup strawberries, chopped
- 1 medium peach, sliced
- 2 cups almond flour
- Pinch of salt

Direction

1. Grease a 7-inch cake pan with butter and line with parchment paper. Set aside.
2. In a bowl, whisk eggs with swerve. Set aside.
3. In a mixing bowl, mix together almond flour, baking powder, and salt.
4. Slowly pour almond flour mixture into the egg mixture and mix constantly.
5. Add the remaining ingredients and fold well.
6. Pour the mixture into the pan and cover the pan with foil.

7. Pour 1 cup of water into the instant pot then place a trivet in the pot.
8. Place cake pan on top of the trivet.
9. Seal instant pot with lid and select manual and set the timer for 25 minutes.
10. Release pressure using the quick release method then open the lid.
11. Remove cake pan from the pot and let it cool completely.
12. Slice and serve.

Nutrition:

Calories 380

Fat 33.6 g

Carbohydrates 12.9 g

Sugar 4.3 g

Protein 12.6 g

Cholesterol 155 mg

Chapter 17. Other Chaffles

48. Basic Keto Low Carb Chaffle Recipe

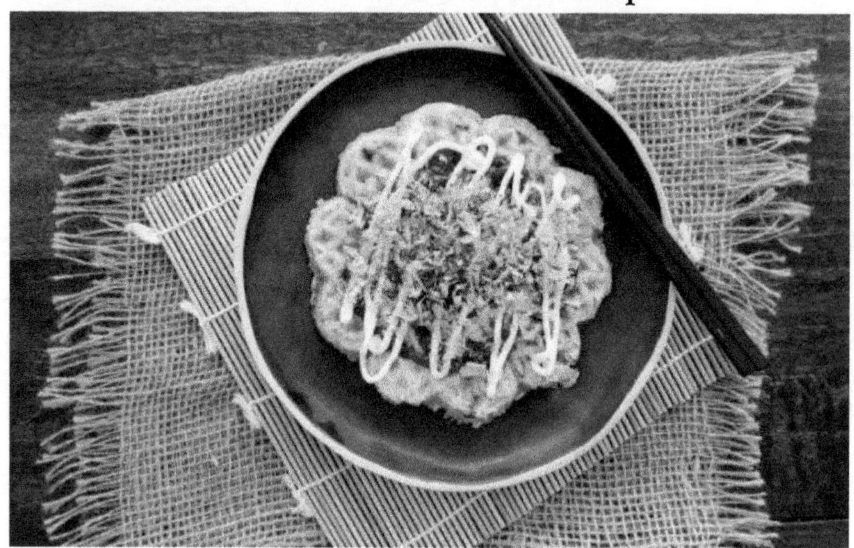

Preparation time: 10 minutes

Cooking Time: 8 Minutes

Servings: 2

Ingredients:

- 1 egg
- 1/2 cup cheddar cheese, shredded

Directions:

1. Turn Chaffle maker on or plug it in so that it heats and grease both sides.
2. In a small bowl, crack an egg, then add the 1/cup cheddar cheese and stir to combine.
3. Pour 1/2 of the batter in the Chaffle maker and close the top.

4. Cooking for 3-minutes or until it reaches desired doneness.
5. Carefully remove from Chaffle maker and set aside for 2-3 minutes to give it time to crisp.
6. Follow the Directions again to make the second chaffle.

Nutrition:

Calories: 58

Fat: 0.4g

Carbohydrates: 0g

Protein: 1.4g

49. Keto Butter Chicken Chaffle with Tzatziki Sauce Recipe

Preparation time: 15 minutes

Cooking Time: 10 minutes

Serving: 2

Ingredients:

- Mozzarella cheese, one cup
- Eggs, two for adding into the chaffles
- Cheddar cheese, one cup
- Salt to taste
- Black pepper to taste
- Almond flour, 17 grams
- Shredded butter chicken, one cup
- Butter chicken sauce, half cup
- Tzatziki sauce, a quarter cup
- Chopped cilantro, 17 grams

Directions:

1. Heat your Chaffle maker.
2. Always remember you heat your Chaffle maker till the point that it starts producing steam.
3. Remove the egg whites in a bowl and beat them to the point that they become fluffy.
4. Beat the egg yolks in a separate bowl.
5. Add in the egg yolks in the egg whites and delicately mix them with a spatula.

6. Combine the eggs and the rest of the ingredients except the chicken, cilantro and tzatziki sauce.
7. Add in the shredded chicken once the rest of the ingredients are well mixed.
8. When your Chaffle maker is heated adequately, pour in the mixture.
9. Close your Chaffle maker.
10. Let your chaffle Cooking for five to six minutes approximately.
11. When your chaffles are done, dish them out.
12. Add the chopped cilantro on top of the chaffles.
13. You can also serve tzatziki sauce alongside your chaffles.
14. Your dish is ready to be served.

Nutrition:

Protein: 31

Fat: 66

Carbohydrates: 2

50. Avocado and Yogurt Chaffles

Preparation time: 10 minutes

Cooking Time: 5 Minutes

Servings: 4

Ingredients:

- 2 cups coconut flour
- 1/2 cup cream cheese, soft
- 1/2 cup yogurt
- 1/2 teaspoon baking soda
- 1 teaspoon baking powder
- 2 tablespoons stevia
- 2 eggs, whisked
- 3 tablespoons coconut oil, melted

Directions:

1. In a bowl, mix the flour with the yogurt and the other ingredients and whisk well.
2. Pour 1/4 of the batter in your Chaffle iron, close and Cooking for 5 minutes.
3. Repeat this with the rest of the batter and serve your chaffles right away.

Chapter 1. Measurement Table

VEGETABLES		
Type	Temperature (Fahrenheit)	Cook Time (Minutes)
Asparagus (sliced)	400	5
Beets (whole)	400	40
Broccoli Florets	400	6
Brussels Sprouts(halved)	380	15
Carrots (sliced)	380	15
Cauliflower florets	400	12
Corn on cob	390	6
Eggplant (cubed)	400	15
Fennel (quartered)	370	15
Green Beans	400	5
Kale leaves	250	12
Mushrooms (sliced)	400	5
Pearl Onions	400	10
Parsnips (cubed)	380	15
Pepper (chunks)	400	15
Small baby potatoes	400	15
Potato (chunks)	400	12

Whole potatoes (baked)	400	40
Squash (chunks)	400	12
Sweet potatoes (baked)	380	30 - 35
Cherry Tomatoes	400	4
Tomatoes (halved)	350	10
Zucchini sticks	400	12

POULTRY		
Type	Temperature (Fahrenheit)	Cook Time (Minutes)
Bone-In breasts	370	25
Boneless breasts	380	12
Drumsticks	370	20
Bone-In thighs	380	22
Boneless thighs	380	18 - 20
Bone-In Legs	380	30
Wings	400	12
Halved Game Hen	390	20
Whole Chicken	360	75
Tenders	360	8 - 10

PORK/LAMB		
Type	Temperature (Fahrenheit)	Cook Time (Minutes)
Loin	360	55
Bone-In Pork Chops	400	12
Tenderloin	370	15
Bacon	400	5 - 7
Bacon	400	6 - 10
Sausages	380	15
Lamb loin chops	400	8 - 12

Measurement Tables

Volume Equivalents (Liquid)

US STANDARD	US STANDARD (OUNCES)	METRIC (APPROXIMATE)
2 tablespoons	1 fl. oz.	30 mL
1/4 cup	2 fl. oz.	60 mL
1/2 cup	4 fl. oz.	120 mL
1 cup	8 fl. oz.	240 mL
11/2 cups	12 fl. oz.	355 mL
2 cups or 1 pint	16 fl. oz.	475 mL
4 cups or 1 quart	32 fl. oz.	1 L
1 gallon	128 fl. oz.	4 L

Volume Equivalents (Dry)

US STANDARD	METRIC (APPROXIMATE)
1/8 teaspoon	0.5 mL
1/4 teaspoon	1 mL
1/2 teaspoon	2 mL
3/4 teaspoon	4 mL
1 teaspoon	5 mL
1 tablespoon	15 mL
1/4 cup	59 mL
1/3 cup	79 mL
1/2 cup	118 mL
2/3 cup	156 mL
3/4 cup	177 mL
1 cup	235 mL
2 cups or 1 pint	475 mL
3 cups	700 mL
4 cups or 1 quart	1 L

Oven Temperatures

FAHRENHEIT (F)	CELSIUS (C) (APPROXIMATE)
250°F	120°C
300°F	150°C
325°F	165°C
350°F	180°C
375°F	190°C
400°F	200°C
425°F	220°C
450°F	230°C

Chapter 2. 30-Day Meal Plan

Day	Breakfast	Lunch	Dinner
Day-1	Peanut Butter and Jelly Sammich Chaffle	Crunchy Fish and Chaffle Bites	Simple Chicken Cheese Chaffle
Day-2	Peanut Butter Cup Chaffles	Grill Pork Chaffle Sandwich	Jamaican Jerk Chicken Chaffle
Day-3	Chocolaty Chaffles	Chaffle and Chicken Lunch Plate	Healthy Chicken Chaffles
Day-4	Mc Griddle Chaffle	Chaffle Minutes Sandwich	Buffalo Chicken Chaffle
Day-5	Cinnamon Swirl Chaffles	Chicken Zinger Chaffle	Garlic Spicy Chicken Chaffle
Day-6	Raspberries Chaffle	Double Chicken Chaffles	Easy Halloumi Burger Chaffle
Day-7	Garlic and Parsley Chaffles	Chaffles with Zucchini Topping	Healthy Chicken Eggplant Chaffle
Day-8	Scrambled Eggs and a Spring Onion Chaffle	Chaffle with Melted Cheese and Bacon	Ginger Chicken Cucumber Chaffle Roll

Day-9	Egg and Cheddar Cheese Chaffle	Grilled Beefsteak and Chaffle	Carbquik Chaffles
Day-10	Chili Chaffle	Breakfast Cauliflower Chaffles and Tomatoes	Chicken Jalapeno Chaffle
Day-11	Simple Savory Chaffle	Classic Beef Chaffle	Chicken Stuffed Chaffles
Day-12	Pizza Chaffles	Beef and Tomato Chaffle	Easy Chicken Vegetable Chaffles
Day-13	Simple Chaffle	Classic Ground Pork Chaffle	Cabbage Chicken Chaffle
Day-14	Chaffles Breakfast Bowl	Spicy Jalapeno Popper Chaffles	Chicken Spinach Chaffle
Day-15	Crispy Chaffles with Sausage	Eggnog Chaffles	Chicken BBQ Chaffle
Day-16	Mini Breakfast Chaffles	Cheddar Jalapeno Chaffles	Crispy Fried Chicken Chaffle
Day-17	Crispy Chaffles with Egg and Asparagus	Low Carb Keto Broccoli Cheese Chaffles	Everything Chaffle
Day-18	Coconut Chaffles	Wonderful Chaffles	Cheesy Salmon Chaffles

Day-19	Keto Basil Buns	Nutter Butter Chaffles	Wholesome Keto Chaffles
Day-20	English Muffin	Buttery Rolls	Keto Cajun Shrimp and Avocado Chaffle Recipe
Day-21	Egg-free Coconut Flour Chaffles	Scallion Mozzarella Cream Cheese Chaffle	Pumpkin Chaffle with Cream Cheese Frosting
Day-22	Simple Chaffle Toast	Lemony Fresh Herbs Chaffles	Chaffle Bread Pudding With Cranberries
Day-23	Sausage Chaffles	Basil Chaffles	Pumpkin Chaffles
Day-24	Egg and Chives Chaffle Sandwich Roll	Scallion Cream Cheese Chaffle	Keto Pumpkin Cheesecake Chaffle
Day-25	Savory Chaffles Bacon and Jalapeno Chaffles	Chicken Taco Chaffles	Pumpkin Spice Chaffles
Day-26	Cheese Broccoli Chaffles	Crab Chaffles	Keto Blueberry Chaffle
Day-27	Bacon and Ham Chaffle	Bacon and Egg Chaffles	Sweet Keto Chaffles

Day-28	Ham and Jalapenos Chaffle	Chicken and Bacon Chaffles	Easy Keto Sandwich Bowl
Day-29	Crispy Bagel Chaffle	Chaffle Katsu Sandwich	Open-Faced Grilled Ham and Cheese Sandwich
Day-30	Sausage and Veggies Chaffles	Pork Rind Chaffles	Cheesy Chaffle Sandwiches with Avocado and Bacon

Conclusion

Ketosis is a metabolic state where the body burns fat rather than glucose (carbohydrates) for fuel. This is due to the lack of glucose in the bloodstream and the absence of insulin (a hormone produced by the pancreas which regulates blood sugar). This metabolic state is known as nutritional ketosis and occurs when the body's fat stores are low enough that it runs out of glycogen (carbohydrates).

The human body accumulates fat to sustain itself. When there are not enough carb stores available to burn, the body will switch over to using fat stores as its primary fuel source. This will continue until there are no more sugar reserves in the general system.

Ketogenic is a low-carb diet that has been proven to burn fat, increase endurance, boost metabolism, and improve overall health. It is a diet that even people who have never tried it have heard of. Ketogenic is so popular because it does so much good for the body, and in such a short time

What are the benefits of having a keto chaffle cookbook? Having the book can help you with your everyday life. You'll have all the recipes you need right at hand. This book will help you achieve your goals faster and will make your life easier to organize. It will also help saving money because you won't have to buy all your ingredients again, which saves money for yourself and helps the environment because you won't be throwing away uneaten food either.

Lightning Source UK Ltd.
Milton Keynes UK
UKHW020657240521
384264UK00005B/158